Health and Optimism

Health and Optimism

Christopher Peterson

Lisa M. Bossio

THE FREE PRESS
A Division of Macmillan, Inc.
NEW YORK
Collier Macmillan Canada
TORONTO
Maxwell Macmillan International
NEW YORK OXFORD SINGAPORE SYDNEY

The Free Press
A Division of Macmillan, Inc.
866 Third Avenue, New York, N.Y. 10022

Collier Macmillan Canada, Inc.
1200 Eglinton Avenue East
Suite 200
Don Mills, Ontario M3C 3N1

Printed in the United States of America

printing number
1 2 3 4 5 6 7 8 9 10

Library of Congress Cataloging-in-Publication Data

Peterson, Christopher.
    Health and optimism / Christopher Peterson, Lisa M. Bossio.
        p. cm.
    Includes bibliographical references and index.
    ISBN 0-02-924981-3
    1. Health.   2. Optimism—Health aspects.   3. Thought and thinking.
    4. Health behavior.   I. Bossio, Lisa M.   II. Title.
    RA776.P4675 1991   90-21244
    613—dc20   CIP

We dedicate this book to our parents,
Robert and Mary Bossio,
Duane and Leota Peterson,
with all of our love.

Contents

Preface

The impetus for this book was a study that one of us (CP) conducted with Martin Seligman and George Vaillant, in which we found that an optimistic way of explaining the causes of bad events—ascertained in a sample of young adult men–predicted their health status 35 years later. We knew the study was intriguing, and we knew it was important in a theoretical sense for showing that psychological states have something to do with physical health.

What we failed to anticipate was the incredible popular interest that the study would generate. Articles about it appeared in magazines across the country and around the world, and they are still doing so.

We enjoyed doing the interviews, and we enjoyed seeing the articles. But research showing that optimism is linked to good health and pessimism to poor health has continued to accumulate. Eventually we felt the need to examine the connections in more detail, to tell the full story ourselves, both more cautiously *and* more optimistically than the writers with whom we talked. Hence this book.

CP is a psychologist who teaches at the University of Michigan. LMB is a free-lance writer and editor who works in the San Francisco Bay Area. We have collaborated on previous projects, and this book seemed a particularly good way to meld our interests and abilities. What you read here is not "as told to" a writer by a researcher. Instead, we worked together in planning and writing every sentence. We have kept several overnight mail businesses profitable for the last year, as drafts winged their way back and forth across the country.

One point of confusion about our collaboration may be apparent, and this is our decision to use the plural pronoun "we" throughout the book, even when describing studies that technically only one of us worked on. We trust that readers will accommodate this usage, because it makes the text flow better.

Research is not done in isolation from other people, and we acknowledge a tremendous debt to many other individuals. Their names are scattered throughout the book, and we thank them collectively here.

And writing is not done in isolation from other people. We thank Albert Cain, Psychology Department Chair at Michigan, for directing Laura Wolff, then the Free Press Senior Editor, to us. We thank Laura for her help in focusing the thesis of the book. Elusive references were provided by Albert Cain, Nancy Cantor, Peter Ditto, and Susan Nolen-Hoeksema. Phil Blumberg made helpful comments on an early draft. Finally, we thank Susan Milmoe, the Free Press Director of Behavioral Sciences and Psychiatry, for her careful and consistent editing.

C. P.—Ann Arbor, MI
L. M. B.—Petaluma, CA

Optimism

The idea does not belong to the
soul; it is the soul that belongs to
the idea.

— *C. S. Peirce*

Over the last fifteen years or so,
Americans have become increasingly health-conscious. Many of us
now believe that our lifestyle may predispose us to illness, disability,
and early death. The media, in responding to this trend, have overwhelmed us with facts and figures about alcohol abuse, smoking, diet,
exercise, toxic waste, and countless other issues and practices. By examining the healthy and unhealthy aspects of ourselves and our communities, we have become more intelligent and more inquisitive,
willing to believe that health is determined in numerous ways.

This new consciousness concerning health entails recognition of
the possibility that psychological states somehow influence our physical well-being. This book describes what is known about the influence
of one such psychological state—optimism—on health. But we must
first define what we mean by optimism. Not everyone feels positively
about thinking positively, and we must clear up some areas of potential misunderstanding.

Optimism has frequently been seen as the philosophy of the fool
and pessimism as the badge of the intellectual (see Table 1–1). The
optimist is out of touch with reality; the pessimist is the sensible one,
able to see the world as it really is.

Mockery of optimism dates at least to the eighteenth century

TABLE 1–1. *Historical Perspective on Optimism Versus Pessimism*

Just how have optimism and pessimism been viewed in the past? Barlett's *Familiar Quotations* and similar sources provide the following:

Optimism . . . is a mania for maintaining that all is well when things are going badly.

—Voltaire (1759)

The basic of optimism is sheer terror.

—Oscar Wilde (1891)

The man who is a pessimist before forty-eight knows too much; if he is an optimist after it, he knows too little.

—Mark Twain (1902)

Optimism: the doctrine or belief that everything is beautiful, including what is ugly, everything good, especially the bad, and everything right that is wrong.

—Ambrose Bierce (1906)

A pessimist is one who has been intimately acquainted with an optimist.

—Elbert Hubbard (1911)

Pessimism, when you get used to it, is just as agreeable as optimism.

—Enoch Arnold Bennett (1918)

American life is a powerful solvent. It seems to neutralize every intellectual element, however tough and alien it may be, and to fuse it with native good will, complacency, thoughtlessness, and optimism.

—George Santayana (1920)

The place where optimism most flourishes is a lunatic asylum.

—Havelock Ellis (1923)

The optimist proclaims that we live in the best of all possible worlds, and the pessimist fears this is true.

—James Branch Cabell (1926)

an optimist is a guy
that has never had
much experience

—Donald Marquis (1927)

Pessimism is only the name that men of weak nerves give to wisdom.

—Bernard De Voto (1935)

What passes for optimism is often the effect of an intellectual error.

—Raymond Aron (1957)

publication of Voltaire's novel *Candide*. One of the characters, the annoying Dr. Pangloss, repeatedly tells the reader that all is for the best in this best of all possible worlds. Voltaire's purpose in *Candide* was to argue against unquestioningly accepting the status quo,[1] but in creating Dr. Pangloss, he unfortunately linked optimism with foolishness.

Those who are truly optimistic are not foolish. Instead, optimism has been systematically misrepresented and indeed caricatured. Consider the American successor to Dr. Pangloss: Pollyanna. It is worth spending some time discussing the Pollyanna phenomenon, because it exemplifies the problems that arise when optimism is conceived in an overly narrow way.

Pollyanna

All that most people know about Pollyanna is that calling someone a "Pollyanna" is an effective way to curb his or her enthusiasm about some future endeavor. Here is the rest of the story. In 1913, an author named Eleanor Porter introduced her in a book called *Pollyanna*.[2] No more than eight pages into the novel, one is struck by the abundance of misfortune in Pollyanna's short life. Her mother has been dead for some time; her father (a penniless minister) has just died himself. As a result, the local Ladies' Aid Society ships Pollyanna from her small western town to New England. Here, she is to live with her only remaining relative, a reclusive Victorian aunt, who is unwelcoming, to say the least. The aunt hated Pollyanna's father because he took her sister away from the family and a wealthy, more likeable suitor. But feeling a sense of duty, she reluctantly takes Pollyanna into her home.

To everyone she meets, Pollyanna explains "the glad game" that her father taught her before he died. He believed that no matter what happens, there is always something to be glad about; one should always hunt for the positive aspects in seemingly bad experiences. In fact, the more catastrophes one faces, the more fun the glad game becomes, because it thereby becomes all the more challenging.

For instance, Pollyanna admits that she misses her father, but she is *glad* that he is dead because he can be in heaven with her mother, the angels, and God. And even though Aunt Polly gives her an ugly attic room with no pictures or rugs or mirrors, she is *glad* for it. If she had a pretty bedroom, she probably wouldn't notice the beautiful trees and houses outside her window. And had her aunt given her a mirror, she would only have to look at her freckles.

Pollyanna plays the glad game with others, but they do not necessarily play along. In fact, her game is often played at the expense of their feelings. When a man breaks his leg walking down the street, Pollyanna is right there to remind him that he should be *glad* that he broke only one leg and not two. Further, he should feel *glad* that he is not a centipede because such a serious fall might have broken fifty legs. She also subjects a depressed invalid, Mrs. Snow, to the glad game. As a literal captive, this poor woman has to listen to Pollyanna say: "I thought—how glad you could be—that other folks weren't like you—all sick in bed like this, you know."[3] And Mrs. Snow should also be *glad* she does not have rheumatic fever, which would limit her ability to move around in bed. Pollyanna tells the gardener, who is complaining about his bent back, that he should feel *glad* about it. After all, he does not have to stoop as far to do his weeding because he's already part way there.

Towards the end of the book, Pollyanna suffers a serious car accident, and her legs become paralyzed. Her reaction, for once, seems realistic. She is grief-stricken and recognizes that it is easier to tell other invalids to feel good about their plight than to tell oneself the same thing. And she admits that the game is not fun if it really *is* hard to play.

But she is determined to find a reason to feel good about her paralysis. And she succeeds. She decides she is *glad* that she cannot walk because her accident has caused Aunt Polly to soften up enough to call her "dear" a lot. And the townspeople suddenly begin to love her. As Aunt Polly explains it to Pollyanna:

> "The whole town is playing the game, and the whole town is wonderfully happier—and all because of one little girl who taught the people a new game, and how to play it."
>
> Pollyanna clapped her hands.
>
> "Oh, I'm so glad," she cried. Then, suddenly, a wonderful light illuminated her face. "Why Aunt Polly, there *is* something I can be glad about, after all. I can be glad I've *had* my legs, anyway—else I couldn't have done—that!"[4]

Of course, the local doctor knows of another doctor who can cure Pollyanna. So, the book ends with her walking her first six steps since the accident . . . and everyone lives gladly ever after.

The story of Pollyanna illustrates the popular conception of blind optimism. Because her game is played for all unfortunate events, it shows no sensitivity to the particular person or situation. Optimists may be viewed, like Pollyanna, as unrealistic people, who spend their time telling others how they *should* feel about the misfortunes in their lives.

To be sure, many Pollyannas mean well, but they still fall short of actually cheering anyone up. An unflagging optimist may find herself taking care of a relative who has cancer. Her loved one may be dying, obviously looking and feeling worse as time passes. But the caretaker says things like "You're doing great" or "I think you're looking better and better each day." The patient knows the truth and finds the constant cheerfulness that bombards him to be inhibiting.

This is not an idle example. A recent survey of cancer patients found that the majority of individuals felt that trite pep talks, however well intended, only made them feel isolated, unable to air their true feelings in an open discussion.[5] The patients wanted to talk about their frustrations and pain and loneliness and anger and fear: all of their "bad" feelings. The caretakers wanted to play the glad game, in effect implying that the patients should suppress their actual emotions. Many patients even began to question whether or not their honest reactions were wrong, as if there is a set of "right" feelings that accompany cancer.

Another survey of cancer patients asked them what *they* considered to be most helpful on the part of friends and family.[6] Love, support, and concern were cited by many patients, along with practical help such as providing transportation. The most frequently mentioned form of support was "just being there."

The Reaction to Pollyanna

Although *Pollyanna* was published without fanfare, the public reaction to it was both swift and dramatic. The book was an overwhelming success, selling over a million copies, and was eventually translated into a dozen languages. Eleanor Porter was bombarded with fan letters from all over the world. Many told of their newly formed Pollyanna Glad Clubs, with various slogans, badges, and buttons. Here are some of the letters:[7]

• A New York Stock Exchange broker suggested to other Stock Exchange members that they read *Pollyanna* aloud to their families.

- A missionary from East India sent the author a photograph of his Indian Glad Girls in their saris.
- An 89-member Glad Club in Scotland wrote Porter that their number one model was Pollyanna. (Florence Nightingale placed second.) Their slogan was: "Be Glad, Be Good, Be Brave."
- Inmates in a state penitentiary called themselves The Pollyanna Glad Kids. These "Kids" were anywhere from 32 to 76 years old. The founder wrote: "Until I came to know Pollyanna and learned to play the Glad Game, I was inclined to be discouraged. I know of a number of men here that Pollyanna turned from a life of worry and gloom".

Pollyanna clones quickly appeared. Fictional characters like Mary Carey and Molly Make-Believe began to spread their wholesome philosophy of life, because this appeared to be what so many people craved. One critic referred to them as professional sunshine-makers.

Eleanor Porter died in 1920, but her character lived on. Two other writers—Harriet Lummis Smith and Elizabeth Borton—continued the series of Pollyanna adventures. There was a 1916 stage rendition of *Pollyanna,* performed by Patricia Collinge. The famous silent-screen star, Mary Pickford, followed in a 1920 film portrayal of the glad girl. And Hayley Mills, of Walt Disney Studios, played Pollyanna in a 1960 movie. The list goes on. Today, a musical based on the Pollyanna story, with an all-black cast, is reportedly in the works.[8]

Even in the beginning, not all readers were smitten with Pollyanna. She raised the hackles of skeptics, who had a heyday with her. Our favorite example is a cartoon from years ago showing a young female lying in the street, a victim of an auto accident. Trapped under the wheels of the car, she cries: "I'm so *glad* it was a limousine!"

Some writers felt that blind optimism was responsible for at least some of America's problems in the twentieth century: the 1929 Wall Street Crash and subsequent depression, for example, in which Pollyanna was identified as a prime scapegoat.[9] It was precisely *because* of our blind optimism that we had overextended our economy, only to find ourselves eating in soup kitchens. Our current national debt, our destruction of the environment, and our nuclear arsenal may indeed reflect blind optimism, as well.

Optimism is still caricatured. For example, the January 1986 issue of *Seventeen* magazine contained a quiz entitled "Are you a Pollyanna or a pessimist?"[10] The quiz posed ten questions, like:

2. Crossword puzzles? You

    a. Do them in pencil.
    b. Do them in ink.
    c. Never try 'em—too hard!

Your choice dictated which category you fell into. You were either a Levelheaded Realist (choice a), a Pollyanna (choice b), or a Melancholy Baby (choice c). Note how "optimism" was juxtaposed not only with pessimism but with levelheaded realism.

Pollyanna in Context

Pollyanna did not appear out of thin air. She can be placed in a tradition of pop psychology: simple formulas that promise health, wealth, and peace of mind for the person who simply thinks the right thoughts. In *The Positive Thinkers,* Donald Meyer traces the history of these promises. Despite many obvious differences, Phineas Quimby, Mary Baker Eddy, Dale Carnegie, Henry Ford, Norman Vincent Peale, and Oral Roberts all fit into this long tradition.[11]

When Eleanor Porter created Pollyanna, she was not inventing the philosophy that her heroine exemplified. She was simply symbolizing it, clearly and effectively. Blind optimism has always found adherents in America, because it is compatible with many of our dominant ideologies: capitalism, laissez-faire politics, and the celebration of individuality.

Who endorses blind optimism? A curious coalition, at least on the face of it: those who already have everything and those who have absolutely nothing. In the former case, the Panglossian view that this is the best of all possible worlds serves to justify the status quo as desirable—as how it *should* be. In the latter case, fantasy is the only route that a truly demoralized person can envision to a better life. That those who play state lotteries tend to be precisely those who cannot afford to do so is another sad example of this tendency.

Neither group's espousal of "optimism" reflects the true meaning of the concept. Optimism is neither political rhetoric nor escapism, though the simplicity of blind optimism explains its enduring appeal in a society addicted to promises of a quick fix. Its effects fail to stand up under close scrutiny, which is why the pop psychologies that Meyer surveyed have been anti-intellectual as well as anti-scientific.

True Optimism Is Complex

According to recent research, optimism offers innumerable benefits: physical health, longevity, professional and personal success. But it is not the optimism of Dr. Pangloss, Pollyanna, or pop psychology that is beneficial; rather, it is an optimism that leads a person to be sensitive to the world on the one hand and active on the other. And even a complex optimism like this is obviously not the only determinant of health, happiness, and success. Many factors besides our expectations affect our health (see Table 1–2).[12] The message from researchers is subtle, but at the same time accurate and credible: optimism is *one of the factors* determining our well-being. We find this exciting enough, particularly because we can sketch some likely ways in which this influence takes place.

How do we approach optimism and its relationship to physical well-being? We start by avoiding "nothing but" analyses. In order to understand a complex phenomenon, scientists and laypeople alike are fond of breaking it into components, and then elevating one component to primary status. Next, they argue that the phenomenon of concern is nothing but whatever it is that they have assigned primary status.

It has been variously asserted that the human condition entails

TABLE 1–2. Some Determinants of Longevity

Factors that are associated with a longer as opposed to a shorter life:

- having grandparents who lived past the age of 80
- having parents who lived past the age of 80
- being the first-born in a family
- being "intelligent"
- *not* being overweight
- eating vegetables and fruits
- *not* eating fatty and sweet foods
- *not* smoking
- drinking alcohol moderately
- exercising
- sleeping 6 to 8 hours every night
- having high socioeconomic status
- living in a rural area
- being married
- having at least two close friends

---

nothing but class struggle, nothing but rewards and punishments, nothing but selfish instincts. Best-selling authors claim that health is nothing but diet, nothing but aerobic exercise, nothing but particular thoughts and feelings. The "nothing but" approach is anything but reasonable.

We propose that optimism involves the whole person, influencing all aspects of one's being—mind, body, and spirit, if you will. (The same holds true for pessimism.) At first glance, Pollyanna's "optimistic" game seems to involve all aspects of her personality, but in fact, her game *smothers* the rest of her being. This is why her legacy distorts the concept of optimism.

Optimism or pessimism refers to someone's expectation for what the future holds. The optimist expects things to work out for the best; the pessimist, just the contrary. If anything, Pollyanna is neither an optimist nor a pessimist. She does not look ahead to a brighter future; instead, she just reacts to the misery of the day. And she does not get depressed about the possibility of doom. Indeed, she gets excited by it.

As we see it, true optimism leads to *action*. Often action is difficult. But the self-professed optimist who fails to make an effort is no more optimistic than the "Sunday Christian" is devout. Later in the book, we describe studies suggesting that one of the ways in which optimism translates itself into good health is through mundane behavior (Chapter 6). In other words, the optimist is healthy because she acts in ways to promote health and combat illness. She eats sensibly, exercises regularly, and knows when to say when.

We have all been told that we could avoid colds if we just stayed away from people who sneezed and coughed. Current thinking has moved beyond the simple formula that germs produce illness. Most of us house all sorts of germs. But we only occasionally fall ill. An intriguing possibility is that optimism protects us against disease, while pessimism makes poor health more likely.

Some Qualifications

Optimism is thus defined as a set of beliefs that leads people to approach the world in an active fashion. Later, we will consider the ways in which optimism and pessimism have been investigated. But first, there are some important qualifications to be borne in mind throughout our discussion.

Optimism is not a rigid trait   People are rarely across-the-board optimists or pessimists, once and forever. True, there are a few extreme individuals who can be characterized as one pure type or the other. And researchers have a simplifying tendency to refer to people as optimists or pessimists. But most people are someplace in the middle of the continuum, and their position may vary with the situation in which they find themselves. Someone may be an optimist with respect to his personal relationships and a pessimist at work—or vice versa.

There are two implications of this qualification. The first is that optimism today does not mean optimism tomorrow. It can be eroded, and sometimes pessimism follows in the wake of difficulties. But the second is that pessimism is malleable as well. Pessimists can become optimists (Chapter 7).

Optimism resides in the real world   Optimism is only helpful when it takes into account reality. If a man is four feet ten inches tall and wants to be a professional athlete, it is not helpful for him to say, "I'm going to practice free throws and forward passes." That is not optimistic. It is deluded. Instead he should find the closest stable and enroll in a riding class. That is realistic but at the same time optimistic.

Optimism entails productive activity   Activity does not entail scurrying about in a frenzy. Being active is doing whatever solves problems or accomplishes goals. So, one of the most active things a person can do in some circumstances is to take time out, drink tea, and relax. The critical element is choosing this course of (peaceful) action over others available in light of what one wishes to achieve.

Caution or contemplativeness should not be confused with passivity. Passivity reflects pessimism, not because of its association with stillness, but because of its lack of association with productivity. Passivity involves helplessness, apathy, and brooding. It feeds upon itself, creating more passivity, and making it ever more difficult to act forthrightly.

Optimism is not a panacea   Positive thoughts do not inevitably result in a long and healthy life. They will not guarantee immunity to the common cold, cancer, AIDS, or arthritis. To believe this is to fall into the "nothing but" trap of theorizing. Optimism is more than just a casual slogan, and the human condition is more than just the point of view that someone entertains about it.

Positive Denial and Healthy Illusions

Psychologists and psychiatrists have long encouraged people to "face reality" and accept whatever evil the world presents to them. Denial was thought to reflect repression, and repression was thought to lie at the base of neurosis. In recent years, these ideas have been challenged by research implying that an *unrealistic* approach to life is associated with good health. If true optimism is not at odds with the facts, how does this argument fit with the contention that it can be beneficial to be a trifle out of touch with reality?

According to psychologist Richard Lazarus, a persuasive case can be made for not facing reality, for engaging in what he terms positive denial.[13] To expect things to work out well, even in the face of evidence that they may not, may set into operation processes which will work against the odds.

Lazarus arrived at his position from studies of how patients respond to severe illness. In some cases, the immediate denial that a disease is severely debilitating can be healthy, because it allows the individual to face her crisis slowly, mobilizing resources at her own speed. Positive denial sustains hope and keeps morale high, which in turn helps her to cope and regain her health.[14] Hackett and Cassem, for example, have demonstrated that people's early denial of serious danger in an episode of myocardial infarction (MI) is associated with lessened mortality.[15]

Of course, there remains a dark side to denial. If taken to an extreme, the person who denies the severity of his illness may not seek or follow the appropriate treatment. Hackett and Cassem have found precisely this problem with denial later on in a person's recovery from MI. Although a firm rule is difficult to specify, it seems that denial is beneficial in the short run when it reduces the individual's anxiety, but not in the long run when it hampers his rehabilitation.

Taylor and Brown have proposed a similar idea in terms of what can be called healthy illusions.[16] By all sorts of criteria of well-being, people are better off if they wear rose-colored glasses. Why not believe that you are a popular and talented person? Why not believe that you have control over the events in your life? Why not believe that everything will work out for the best? There are demonstrable benefits to these beliefs—including the ability to care about others, personal happiness and contentment, creativity, and productivity.

The caution, of course, is that sometimes these notions can be grievously wrong. If one's illusions do more than massage reality, if they actually get in the way of seeing a runaway locomotive, then obviously they are not as benign as Taylor and Brown hypothesize.

The metaphor of rose-colored glasses is attractive because no one suggests that those who don them keep their eyes closed. Positive denial and healthy illusions are useful to the degree that they impart a pleasing tint to the way the world is; anything more, and beware!

Optimism should *not* be equated with positive denial or healthy illusion, although they are all related. There are several important distinctions. First, optimism is reality based, not reality distorting. This idea is apparent in Hackett and Cassem's research on denial among MI patients. It is realistic in one sense to deny difficulties early on because there is nothing to lose by doing so and perhaps something to gain. There is an old argument about why one should believe in God. If God does not exist, then what has it cost you? And if there is a God, can you afford not to believe? Perhaps the point is that the usefulness of these views reduces to a cost-benefit analysis, which is obviously reality based.

Second, many beliefs are neither realistic nor unrealistic, because particular events in one's life may be too singular and too ambiguous to interpret definitively. Some things are more certain than others, and the optimist does not fly in the face of sure things. But if there is some doubt, then why not fill it with hope? It costs little, and it may even pay dividends.

Third, optimism translates itself into actions which change the world and hence change the optimist. It is thus infused with a sense of agency. Positive denial and healthy illusions may do this, but they may also rationalize inactivity.

Optimistic and Pessimistic Thinking

Before we move on to Chapter 2 to discuss the studies that link optimism to good health, we want to describe exactly how we determine that given people are relatively optimistic or pessimistic. This discussion is an important one, because research is only as convincing as the concrete procedures on which it rests. We have tried to go about measuring optimism in a way that does justice to its complexity.

The occasion for thought   Most of us do not think too much about thought. We may take it so much for granted that we overlook some of its most striking characteristics, including the fact that our conscious minds are *not* always engaged. Indeed, much of the time we operate on autopilot, in a state that psychologist Ellen Langer describes as mindlessness.[17]

When we are mindless in the way that Langer defines it, we are neither zombies nor stuporous. Rather, we act smoothly and efficiently, carrying out well-learned routines without devoting conscious attention to their details. Mindlessness becomes an issue only when a well-learned routine fails to work in given circumstances. Consider buying and then driving a new car. Part of this experience, along with the new car smell and the price sticker carefully preserved in the window, is a series of concrete discoveries about how it differs from the old car:

- Ouch! I have to duck my head differently to get in and out.
- *This* switch controls the windshield wipers, and *that* switch controls the lights; no, it's just the opposite.
- The brakes work well.
- Is it possible that there is no volume control on the radio?
- Why can't I pull the key out of the ignition?

One makes these discoveries not by anticipating how the new car differs from the old car but through mistakes that follow from the unquestioned assumption that the two cars are exactly the same.

In the grand scheme, the new car owner of course knows that the cars are different, but his behavior is still mindless. In this mundane sense, he does not know the difference because he quite literally is not thinking. Only gradually, as he is repeatedly jerked into awareness by mistakes, does he replace his old routines with new ones. And when it comes time to replace this car with yet another new car, the process will repeat itself again.

Here then is an important lesson about the occasion for thought. We think—become aware or act mindfully—when we encounter events that surprise us. Other studies by psychologists elaborate this lesson by identifying as occasions for thought events that are unpleasant and/or highly significant.[18] This all makes wonderful sense, and may well have a basis in the evolution of our species. It is highly functional to think in circumstances that are unusual, aversive, or significant. And it may well be functional *not* to think in other circumstances, because we save time and effort by relying on mindless routines adequate to the task at hand.

Implications for research These ideas about the occasion for thought suggest how a researcher might profitably go about investigating optimism and pessimism. Consider the implications of what we have said about the occasion for thought. Optimistic (or pessimistic) thoughts are rarely front and center in people's minds. They are nonetheless present, in an obvious way as well as a less obvious way. The obvious way is that optimistic or pessimistic thoughts occur when we are surprised, disconcerted, or challenged. The less obvious way is that our optimism or pessimism permeates our very routines. An optimistic routine presupposes a good future. Consider what a waitress does when a customer requests change for a twenty. Can an appropriate tip be readily given from what she brings back? If so, the waitress has an optimistic routine. If she brings two fives and a ten, and the meal cost $4.95, she is either crazy or pessimistic (or perhaps both).

People can tell a researcher something of the optimism or pessimism inherent in their thoughts or routines, but they will probably not be perfectly accurate. This is not because they intend to mislead, but because thoughts can sometimes be elusive, particularly those that become woven into mindless routines. What people say about what they think does not always convey what they actually think.[19] We must be cautious in interpreting studies in which people are simply asked if they are optimistic or pessimistic.

One way to avoid some of the problems inherent in asking people to respond about their optimism or pessimism off the tops of their heads is to arrange matters so that they are more likely to be mindful than mindless when responding. A useful approach is to confront people with a bad event, and then ask them to make sense of it.

We have usually studied the psychological states of optimism and pessimism by seeing how people explain the causes of the bad events that befall them. There is extensive psychological literature that concerns itself with how people offer explanations for events. This line of work, in the framework of what is known as attribution theory, shows in a variety of ways that people's interpretations of the causes of events affect their subsequent feelings and actions.[20] There are considerable methodological advantages to studying people's causal explanations (or attributions), because when people explain events, they are usually mindful. Accordingly, their responses are apt to be valid indicators of what and how they think.

Explanatory Style

When people become mindful in the wake of some event, one of the things they often do is to ask, "Why did this happen?" Sometimes reality provides an unequivocal answer:

- I got a speeding ticket because my speedometer is broken.
- I lost my job because the company went bankrupt.
- I flunked the test because I didn't study.
- My marriage broke up because he drank too much.

But sometimes there is ambiguity about the real cause of an event. In these cases, people rely on habitual explanations, what we call their *explanatory style.*[21]

Ickes and Layden provided this striking example from a "Dear Abby" column:

> I am a 34-year old woman who has divorced three husbands. (Not my fault. I always picked losers.)
>
> My problem is my nose. I had plastic surgery on it when I was 18, and the doctor botched the job, so at 21 I had it reshaped and then it was worse. I think it makes me look stuck up and keeps me from making friends.
>
> I went to a well-known plastic surgeon, and I offered to pay him in full in advance but he refused to take me as a patient! He said he didn't think any plastic surgeon could please me because I had "emotional and social problems" I should face instead of blaming everything on my nose. Then he insulted me further by suggesting that I use my money to see a psychiatrist!
>
> Abby, there is nothing wrong with my mind. It's my nose! Will you please recommend a good plastic surgeon? I can afford to go anywhere. *

All other things being equal, people have their own ways of explaining disparate events.

How do we study explanatory style? A person's causal explanations are described along three different dimensions.[22] First, does the attributed cause refer to something about the person offering it or to something about other people or circumstances? This dimension ranges from *internal* causes at one extreme ("it's me") to *external* causes at the other ("it's the economy").

Second, does it refer to something that will last for a long time, or to something that is fleeting? In the former case, the cause is regarded as *stable* ("Why did that happen—I'll tell you why: human nature, plain and simple"). In the latter case, the cause is *unstable* ("I threw the home run pitch because I slipped during my delivery").

*Taken from the Dear Abby column by Abigail Van Buren. Copyright 1976 Universal Press Syndicate. Reprinted with permission. Cited in Ickes and Layden, 1978, p. 119.

Third, does the causal explanation refer to something that leads to a variety of outcomes in a person's life, or to something that only affects the particular event in question? Pervasive explanations are termed *global*. So, "my life is the pits" qualifies as a global cause. Circumscribed explanations are called *specific:* "My boss hates Monday mornings so he refuses to take calls before noon."

We regard explanatory style as a cognitive habit, a way of routinely linking bad events on the one hand with causes on the other. In some cases, it can be described as optimistic. To explain some bad happening as due to factors outside oneself that are neither long-lasting nor pervasive is in effect to say, "It was just one of those things." Whatever produced it is unlikely to be around tomorrow, and positive expectations for the future remain highly plausible. In other cases, explanatory style can be seen as pessimistic. "I'm a wretched and flawed excuse for a human being" has a timeless quality to it.

When someone explains bad events in terms of character flaws, he puts himself at risk for apathy, depression, failure, illness, and even death. Those who blame themselves for bad events *and* feel powerless to change them will find themselves in a particularly stressful situation. Prolonged stress weakens the immune system which in turn makes illness more likely. An optimistic explanatory style makes this chain of events less likely.

Here are some excerpts—appropriately disguised—from a letter one of us received from a former student asking for a letter of recommendation for a job:

> I left town about a week ago. I thought I was ready for marriage—but my persistent fear of someone getting too close to me took over. So I left. My life goes on, but it looks pretty bleak. I just tend to push people away. I'm real bad about that. I always feel embarrassed.
>
> . . . I have hit rock bottom. I cannot find a job other than waiting on tables. I'm doing a lot of soul-searching, and I don't like what I find.
>
> . . . I was wondering if you would mind writing me a letter of recommendation. I feel bad asking you. I always figured you disliked me pretty much. I've been pretty screwed up. I've never faced myself. I'd understand if you just threw this in the trash and told me to forget it.

In contrast, consider these excerpts—not at all disguised—from a story in *Sports Illustrated* about baseball player Gary Carter:

It is a dank, dismal morning . . . a good morning to pull the covers over your head. Mets catcher Gary Carter, 33, opens one eye at 8:30, awaiting the news from his battered body. "I'm feeling pretty good," he thinks. He cautiously moves an arm, a leg and then, the real test, his neck and upper back. "Hey, maybe I really am feeling good."

He risks getting up and is elated: "I am feeling good. I am being rewarded." And why not? In a 13-year career, he has had three knee operations, two broken thumbs, three broken ribs and ligament tears in each ankle. For this season, add a bruised toe, an aching right knee and a nagging back ailment. . . .

Through it all, Carter remains relentlessly happy. "I know some people think my smile is too big," he says. "But all I do is smile and enjoy the game. Is there anything wrong with that?"

Carter won't be playing today, though. He is routinely given a rest when day games follow night games. . . . "Hey," he says, "maybe I'll pinch-hit and win the game."

. . . He isn't needed. The Mets whip the Phillies 8–3.

. . . "Hey, what a great day . . . I didn't make any errors or any outs.

. . . I'd be silly to say every day is a great day, but most of them are. . . . This one was."*

The former student and Gary Carter are doing similar things in these excerpts. Both are describing events in their lives. In the course of describing these events, both are explaining them. And in their explanations, both are consistent within themselves. But for all these similarities, each offers a very different explanation for bad events. The low self-esteem and pessimism of the former student almost leap off the page from her causal explanations. To judge from his public utterances, Carter's self-esteem is highly intact, and it is hard to imagine him having very many pessimistic thoughts even in his most private moments.

Measuring Explanatory Style

Researchers have measured an individual's explanatory style in two ways. The first is with a questionnaire called the Attributional Style Questionnaire (ASQ) that asks people to imagine a series of hypothetical events involving themselves.[23] For example: "You can't get all the work done that your supervisor requires." The respondents then write down the cause they would come up with if this event actually happened. People never have much trouble doing so. Then respondents use three separate rating scales to indicate first the degree to which the cause they wrote down is internal or external, then the degree to which it is stable or unstable, and finally the degree to which it is global or specific (see Table 1–3).

Ratings are averaged across the three dimensions and across the different events of the ASQ to yield an overall score for explanatory style, ranging from pessimistic (internal, stable, and global causes) to

---

TABLE 1–3. *Example of An Attributional Style Questionnaire Item*

Please try to imagine yourself in the situation that follows. If such a situation happened to you, what do you feel would have caused it? While events may have many causes, we want you to pick only one— *the major cause if this event happened to you.*

Please write the cause in the blank provided after each event. Next we want you to answer three questions about the cause you provided. First, is the cause of this event something about you or something about other people or circumstances? Second, is the cause of this event something that will occur in the future or not? Third, is the cause of this event something that affects all situations in your life or something that just affects this type of event?

Event: You cannot get all the work done that your supervisor has assigned.

A. Write down the one major cause: _____

B. Is the cause of this something about you or something about other people or circumstances? (circle one number)

| totally due to others | 1 | 2 | 3 | 4 | 5 | 6 | 7 | totally due to me |

C. In the future, will this cause again be present? (circle one number)

| never present | 1 | 2 | 3 | 4 | 5 | 6 | 7 | always present |

D. Is this cause something that affects just this type of situation, or does it also influence other areas of your life? (circle one number)

| just this situation | 1 | 2 | 3 | 4 | 5 | 6 | 7 | all situations |

---

optimistic (external, unstable, and specific). Studies using this measure find that people respond in a consistent and stable fashion.

The second measure of explanatory style is the more flexible strategy of content analysis. Researchers scrutinize written or spoken material—letters, diaries, autobiographies, interviews in newspapers, psychotherapy transcripts, even graffiti—for any mention of negative events and accompanying explanations. When they have located bad events and their explanations, the researchers rate them for their internality, stability, and globality.

This method is called the CAVE technique, an acronym for Content Analysis of Verbatim Explanations.[24] See Table 1–4 for an example of a letter in which bad events and causal explanations have been highlighted. This is a relatively upbeat letter, despite the bad events that are recounted. The writer's explanations point to external and circumscribed causes. A more pessimistic individual might have explained her failure to write as due to her lack of organization, the chaos at work as resulting from her inability to catch on to routines, and the broken chair as a consequence of her own carelessness.

What is exciting about this approach to studying optimism is that researchers can ascertain someone's characteristic style of thinking after the fact, so long as some written record has been left behind. Thus they can study long-term consequences of optimistic or pessimistic explanatory style not by waiting for decades to see what happens to people, but by "going back" to discover the antecedents of outcomes that are already known.

Explanatory style is not the only indication of someone's characteristic optimism or pessimism. There has been a recent explosion of interest in optimistic and pessimistic thinking, and a number of new research measures are available. We think our measures of explanatory style have particular virtues because the explanations are offered when research subjects are in a mindful state. However, other measures do overlap and often show similar relationships with such outcomes as health and illness. We will discuss these cognates and cousins in Chapter 3.

The important point is that explanatory style is a habit, a way of thinking that people impose on events when all other things are equal. There are times when things are not equal, however, and reality provides a clear answer about the operative cause of an event. Explanatory style is most pertinent to what a person is all about precisely in situations that are ambiguous, when there really are no arguably correct (or incorrect) answers about causes.

In our earlier discussion of Pollyanna, we argued that optimism

TABLE 1–4. *Example of the CAVE Technique*

Dear __,

Let me apologize. *I haven't written in so long. The move and the new job have eaten up so much time.* But things on the whole are going pretty well, and I can't wait to tell you about them.

Work is a challenge, to say the least. *The person in the job before me left things in a shambles.* I think she knew for a while she was going to quit, so *she didn't do any filing for about six months.* I finally got everything in order by working twelve hours a day at it. And you know what I think of filing!

The only thing that was broken in the move was one of the legs on a kitchen chair. Something must have shifted in the U-Haul and crunched it. *The roads in West Virginia can be bumpy.* Everything is now unpacked, and it looks great in my new apartment. I have a lovely view of an orchard.

I hope you can come visit soon. Give my best to everyone. I'll write more later.

Love, __

Bad Event	Cause
not writing	"the move and the new job have eaten up so much time"
things at work were in shambles	"she didn't do any filing for about six months"
broken chair	"the roads in West Virginia can be bumpy"

is reality based. Part of taking into account reality is knowing when there are clear causes and when there are not. When "allowed" to analyze a situation, some people draw on an optimistic view and others on a pessimistic one. To put forward a particular interpretation of events when evidence is to the contrary is to be neither optimistic nor pessimistic, but simply wrong and perhaps even delusional. Remember, Pollyanna did not wear rose-colored glasses so much as she closed her eyes tightly in any and all circumstances.

Explanatory style was not originally formulated as a way to study optimism and its relationship to physical well-being. Rather, it was articulated as a personality trait by researchers interested in depression,[25] who somewhat earlier were interested in how people responded to bad events,[26] and who even earlier were interested in how animals responded to bad events.[27] The phenomenon of interest throughout these investigations is called *learned helplessness.*[28] We discuss learned helplessness in detail in Chapter 5. For more than two decades, researchers have looked at how reactions to bad events are influenced by one's thoughts about these events. Their ideas offer many hints for those of us seeking to understand just how an optimistic outlook might affect health.

CHAPTER

2

Health and Optimism: Establishing the Link

> Pain is inevitable. Suffering
> is optional.
>
> — *M. Kathleen Casey*

Everyone *knows* that psychological
states have something to do with health and illness. We need not look
far for striking examples of people whose good cheer and perseverance allow them to fight off the effects of illness. We can just as easily
find examples of their tragic counterparts: people whose hopelessness
and depression lead them to give up in the face of a physical challenge,
and eventually die.

One of the best-known examples of perseverance in the face of
illness is Norman Cousins's successful fight against a debilitating col-
lagen disease by mustering his positive emotions.[1] And Bernie Siegel's
catalogues of medical miracles have been read and cherished by millions.[2] We find these stories of great interest, but at the same time, we
take a skeptical view. These particular examples prove very little other
than that the course of people's physical health can vary drastically.

They do not demonstrate conclusively that psychological factors
have anything to do with good or bad health. They do not identify
which psychological factors might be critical. They do not allow us to
generalize to other people. We are happy for Norman Cousins that he
is alive, recovered from a life-threatening illness, but we do not know
what else to say about his story.

Perhaps the real value of such striking examples is that they legitimize closer scrutiny of the link between psychological states and physical well-being. Researchers have recently been taking these closer looks, finding indeed that optimism leads to better health than pessimism. One ensuing problem is that these research findings are not so sensational as the striking examples. The careful generalizations offered by a researcher do not have the same impact as the story of a particular person with a particular outlook who recovered from a particular disease that threatened his life. But the researchers, unlike the storytellers, attempt to identify active causes. They are alert to alternative explanations. Their studies pass the test of science.

The ideal investigation of the psychological precursors of illness should satisfy procedural criteria such as these:

1. *The research design must be longitudinal.* Research participants must be followed over time. Merely showing a contemporaneous association between psychological states and physical health or illness leaves unanswered the direction of the implied effect. Perhaps illness or health determines one's psychological state. Or perhaps some other factor, appropriately called a "third variable" by researchers, gives rise to both the psychological state on focus and one's health status.

2. *Any longitudinal design must span enough time for change in health to take place.* This may require several years or even decades. Because we are exploring new territory, we are not quite sure what the right time frame should be. We must therefore be leery of researchers who report "no results" from their studies trying to link psychological states with health and illness. Perhaps there really is no link to be found, and the researchers indeed were on a wild goose chase. But perhaps the optimal time span was not chosen. In this chapter, we will describe studies with positive results, and we accord considerable status to these findings.[3]

3. *The initial health status of the research participants must be known when the investigation begins.* There is no point in finding that sick people stay sick, while healthy people stay healthy. Many researchers start with people's current health status and then try to work backwards to reconstruct what they were like in the first place. This is a reasonable procedure if the distant past can be reconstructed with accuracy, but that is not easy to do. People distort their past, innocently or otherwise, and may retrospectively make better sense of what ensued than the facts warrant. Sick people may tell a story that

rationalizes their sickness, as healthy people may rationalize their health.

4. *An adequate number of research participants must be studied* because links between psychological states and illness—if they exist—are apt to be subtle in nature and thus modest in strength. Only with a large number of research participants can patterns be discerned and third variables ruled out. Case studies of single individuals, no matter how striking, can be scientifically ambiguous precisely on this score.

5. *The psychological states of interest must be well defined and able to be measured in a reliable and valid fashion.* Researchers should avoid in particular measures that are contaminated by a person's health status—which means that they end up using one aspect of his health to predict another aspect, so of course these will be related but will prove nothing. This has been a problem in stress research, for instance, where "illness" is considered a stressful life event that ends up being related to subsequent illness.

6. Similarly, *objective measures of health and illness must be made* at the time that an investigation begins, during the study, and at the time at which it ends. Health and illness may seem easy for a researcher to ascertain. But the more closely they are examined, the fuzzier they become. Many criteria for physical illness have been employed by researchers:

- complaints of feeling ill
- the presence of particular symptoms such as swollen glands
- the diagnosis of particular illnesses by examining physicians
- the corroboration of diagnoses by blood tests, urine tests, X-rays, and the like
- bodily responses like immune functioning that show how the body responds to siege
- total lifespan
- survival as opposed to death

Some of these criteria seem more objective than others, but there is fuzziness even in the criterion of death. A tongue-in-cheek article in a public health journal pointed out that because the legal definition of death varies from state to state—for example, cessation of brain activity in New Jersey versus cessation of cardiac function in New York—people are "dead" or not depending on where they happen to find themselves. Resurrection may be possible, depending on the direction the paramedics happen to be driving!

Knowing that no particular criterion is foolproof, researchers nonetheless must settle on a strategy for measuring health status. Perfect agreement among the various criteria of illness is not to be found. There are people who "feel" fine but have critical illnesses; there are people who "feel" poorly but show great vigor. There are diseases without symptoms, symptoms without diseases. One of the best established findings in the twentieth century is that morbidity (illness) and mortality (death) do not perfectly line up once we look separately at males and females.[4] Women have more illnesses than men, but they also live longer.[5]

Untouched in any of these research definitions is what it means to be healthy. Most researchers adopt the convention of regarding health as the absence of illness, defined in any of the possible ways that it might be defined. This is less than ideal, and we will return to the topic of how best to characterize optimal living in Chapter 8.

Science and Generalizations

Despite the difficulties inherent in this research, well-conducted studies support the conclusion that people with optimistic beliefs experience better health than those with pessimistic beliefs. But there will be exceptions, because these statements are necessarily generalizations. The exceptions do not disprove the generalization, so long as the contrary examples are in the minority.

Consider Gilda Radner, the comedienne who recently died of ovarian cancer. In her life, she exemplified many of the qualities that researchers (and everyday people) link to good health and long life.[6] She was cheerful; she was optimistic; she had supportive friends and family; she was a problem solver. But she died at an early age, her cancer undetected until its later stages. Her story is a somber reminder that scientific studies offer us generalizations and not guarantees.

What generalizations can be offered about optimism and health? We will describe half a dozen studies that have specifically addressed this relationship.

A Thirty-Five-Year Longitudinal Study
of Optimism and Health

The Harvard Study of Adult Development began when the William T. Grant Foundation funded a project to study "the kinds of people who are well and do well."[7] This ongoing longitudinal investigation was initiated in 1937 by Clark Heath and Arlie Bock at the Harvard University Health Sciences and is now directed by George E. Vaillant of Dartmouth Medical School. It represents a unique source of data about human growth and development across the lifespan. The Harvard Study has allowed researchers to make important statements about coping[8] and alcoholism.[9] It has also allowed an exemplary study of optimism and its relationship to health to be carried out.

The study began with physically healthy, mentally healthy, and successful members of the Harvard classes of 1942 through 1944. Potential research subjects were first screened on the basis of academic success (40% of the entire student body was excluded), then on the basis of physical and psychological health (another 30% was excluded), and finally on the basis of nominations by college deans of the most independent and accomplished individuals. In all, 268 young men were included in the study.

Each subject, while an undergraduate, underwent an extensive physical examination and completed a battery of personality and intelligence tests. After graduation, the subjects completed annual questionnaires about their employment, family, health, and so on. Periodic physical examinations of each subject were conducted by his own doctor. Only ten men withdrew from the study during college, and two more after graduation.

The Harvard Study of Adult Development is a very special investigation because it satisfies most of the criteria for an ideal study of how psychological states might influence physical health. It is longitudinal; it has a large number of research participants; it has low attrition; it has good measures of physical health—i.e., physician examinations buttressed with medical tests.

The study also makes it possible for us to ascertain the characteristic optimism or pessimism of the research participants when they were young. Among the many measures completed by subjects was a questionnaire they responded to in 1946 that was open-ended and asked about difficult wartime experiences:

> What difficult personal situations did you encounter (we want details), were they in combat or not, or did they occur in relations with superiors or men under you? Were these battles you had to fight within yourself? How successful or unsuccessful in your own opinion were you in these situations? How were they related to your work or health? What physical or mental symptoms did you experience at such times?

These questions are an invitation to be mindful, and research participants certainly were. Their answers to these questions were more essays than brief statements—always articulate and sincere, sometimes poignant, and sometimes passionate.[10]

One of us (CP) planned and conducted an investigation of the explanatory style of these men, with psychologist Martin Seligman from the University of Pennsylvania and psychiatrist George Vaillant at Dartmouth Medical School.[11] We chose an arbitrary subset of 99 subjects, and we read through their 1946 essays to find causal explanations of bad events. For the 99 men, we found a total of 1102 bad events and causal explanations, an average of 11.1 per research subject.

Four research assistants rated these causal explanations as described in the previous chapter, according to their internality (versus externality), stability (versus instability), and globality (versus specificity). Our four judges agreed well with each other about how to rate particular causal explanations, which means that the procedure was reliable.

We then combined the ratings by averaging across the judges, across the three rating dimensions, and finally across the different events explained by a particular research subject. What resulted was a set of 99 scores, one per subject, that placed each someplace along the dimension ranging from an extremely optimistic explanatory style to an extremely pessimistic one.

Along the way to assigning a single optimism-pessimism score to each research subject, we lingered long enough to calculate whether a given individual explained events in a consistent fashion. Remember our earlier cautions that sometimes the reality of events dictates how they are explained, thus precluding someone's habitual view of things from affecting given explanations. This might mean that our scores reflected the particular wartime events encountered by a subject (reality) and not the way he habitually thought about such events (explanatory style). Our check on consistency allayed this fear about the validity of our procedure.

Research subjects indeed explained disparate events in the same way. Those who were optimistic about a particular event tended as well to be optimistic about a second, third, or fourth. Similarly, those who were pessimistic in the way they explained one event were also pessimistic in the way they explained other events. See Table 2–1 for representative explanations by an especially optimistic research subject and by an especially pessimistic one.

We have detailed how the habitual level of optimism of our research subjects was ascertained. Now let us turn to the assessment of

TABLE 2–1. *Optimistic and Pessimistic Explanations
(Harvard Study)*

Explanations for bad events offered by one of the most optimistic individuals in this study:

"I caught pneumonia [because] . . . I returned to a colder climate."
"I was unhappy at work [because] . . . many things were left undone in the press of circumstances."
"I was in danger during the aerial attack [because] . . . I was not assigned to a specific task which kept me in a single position."

Explanations for bad events offered by one of the most pessimistic individuals in this study:

"I was not happy in the service [because of my] . . . intrinsic dislike for the military."
"I dislike work [because there is] . . . no room for anything else—nor can plans be made."
"I'm not married [because] . . . I have no prospects."

---

their physical health. At eight times in a research subject's life—at ages 25 (approximately when the open-ended questionnaire we just described was completed), 30, 35, 40, 45, 50, 55, and 60, his personal physician completed a thorough physical exam and forwarded the results to a research internist at the Harvard Study. The doctor—obviously unaware of the research subject's optimism or pessimism, because these were not to be ascertained until years later—then rated each subject in light of the exam results in the following way:

1 = good health, normal
2 = multiple minor complaints, mild back trouble, prostatitis, gout, kidney stones, single joint problems, chronic ear problems
3 = probably irreversible chronic illness without disability; illness that will not fully remit and will probably progress—like treated hypertension, emphysema with cor pulmonae, diabetes
4 = probably irreversible chronic illness with disability—for example, myocardial infarction with angina, disabling back trouble, hypertension *and* extreme obesity, diabetes *and* severe arthritis, multiple sclerosis
5 = deceased

From age 50 on, the research internist also had available blood and urine tests, an electrocardiogram, and a chest X-ray for most of the research subjects.[12] Table 2–2 gives the mean scores for these health ratings at the different ages in life.

One more measure was available for each subject. In 1945, a global rating was made by an examining psychiatrist who attempted to predict the individual's likelihood of encountering emotional difficulties in the future. This is important to know about each subject because we would want to rule out the possibility that an underlying emotional difficulty—depression, for instance—might cause both a pessimistic worldview and poor physical health.

Not surprisingly, as subjects became older, their health on the whole worsened. However, what also happened was that the *range* of scores increased. In other words, there was an ever greater difference between the most and least healthy. This trend in and of itself is hardly unexpected, because all subjects started out as extremely healthy. Remember the stringent selection criteria. But what is interesting is that even for extremely healthy young men, some became quite sickly as they aged. Of the 99 men we studied, 13 died before age 60. Our appetite was whetted for discovering what might make the difference between those with a good outcome and those without. Would optimism be relevant?

Our procedure was complex. Our results in contrast are quite simple. Overall, men who used optimistic explanations for bad events at age 25 were healthier later in life than men who offered pessimistic explanations. This correlation held even when their initial physical

TABLE 2–2. *Mean Scores on Health Status Measure (Harvard Study)*

Age	*Physical health rating*	*Number deceased*
25	1.16	0
30	1.20	0
35	1.30	0
40	1.41	2
45	1.60	4
50	1.91	5
55	2.21	9
60	2.67	13

Source: Peterson, Seligman, and Vaillant (1988).

and emotional soundness were taken into account by the appropriate statistical machinations. So, *optimism early in life is associated with good health later in life.*

To be more specific about these important findings,[13] optimism was unrelated to health at ages 30 through 40, but thereafter the relationship emerged. It reached its most robust level at age 45, approximately 20 years after the time that explanatory style was assessed. Thereafter, the relation between optimism and health fell off somewhat.

We also looked at how optimism (at age 25) was associated with *changes* in a subject's health status from one age to another. This lets us zero in on exactly where optimism starts to have benefits (and pessimism costs). To some degree, pessimism was associated with a worsening of health from ages 35 to 40. But the link became abundantly clear between ages 40 and 45. Here those who were optimistic as youths maintained their health, in contrast to those who were pessimistic. These latter individuals showed a marked deterioration.

Associations between variables (like optimism and health) are often described with statistics termed correlation coefficients. The larger the correlation coefficient, the stronger the relationship it describes—the more the one variable is associated with the other. The correlation coefficients we obtained between early optimism and later health were as high as .37. But what does this really mean? Correlation coefficients have no intuitive meaning to most people, including trained researchers.[14]

There is little chance that our patterns were flukes. Indeed, some of the patterns we found in the data would arise by chance fewer than one time out of a thousand, so we know that the results are solid— what statisticians call statistically significant. At the same time, there was not a one-to-one relationship between optimism and pessimism on the one hand and good and poor health on the other. While it is an accurate generalization to say that the optimists were healthier than the pessimists, there also were exceptions: optimists who died young and pessimists who stayed alive and well.

The strengths of our relationships fall into a range of what statisticians refer to as "moderate" correlations. Interestingly, some other well-known and well-accepted relationships involving health status— for example, the one between cigarette smoking and the development of lung cancer—are not as robust as the one we discovered in this study.

Optimism did not predict immediate health status. This is not surprising because in our sample there was little variation in health to begin with. But by early middle age (35–50), health became more variable, and psychological factors began to play a role.[15] In later middle age (50–60), the relationship between optimism and health fell off a bit. We have as yet no good explanation for this, but we suspect that constitutional factors or lifestyle or both start to exert dominant influences on health at this time.

Any research study, no matter how striking its results, falls short of being the final word on a topic. A major shortcoming of the study we have just described is, of course, that its sample was originally chosen *not* to be representative of the population as a whole. This does not detract from the value of the study as a demonstration. Yes, under some circumstances for some people, psychological states are related to health. But questions arise about the boundary conditions. Does the relationship hold for all people in all circumstances? Generalizing from the very special participants in the study is obviously a problem. These were initially healthy, often wealthy, successful men, mostly from the northeast United States.

It is a standard joke among researchers that the one conclusion that always follows from every study ever done is that "more research is needed." This is no less true in the present case. We must establish broadly the link between a person's explanatory style and his or her health in order to address the problem of limited generality of results from the Harvard Study. In the remainder of this chapter, we describe other studies that further support this correlation.

A Study of Optimism and the Common Cold

Another investigation of the relationship between explanatory style and physical health used a different population of research subjects, a different time frame, a different measure of optimism and pessimism, and two different criteria for good versus poor health.[16] It qualifies as a conceptual replication of the study just described. It tests the same hypothesis as the other study, but it does so with different procedures.

This study began during the fall of 1984, what we refer to as Time One. Our research subjects were 172 undergraduates at Virginia Tech, in Blacksburg, Virginia. They completed a version of the Attributional Style Questionnaire, described in the previous chapter. This measured their habitual use of optimistic versus pessimistic explanations for bad events.

They also completed a measure we dubbed the Illness Scale, a questionnaire that asked them to describe all the illnesses they had experienced during the previous 30 days.[17] For each illness, the research subjects described the date that the symptoms were first noticed and the date that they were last present. The degree of illness can then be calculated as the number of different days during the month that at least one symptom was present. Scores range from 0 to 30, and the higher the score, the more "ill" we say the individual was.

The impossibility of perfectly measuring health and illness was noted earlier. The Illness Scale has its flaws. There are people who become acutely ill, on the doorstep of death itself, whose symptoms go away within two days. There are also people with lingering but trivial colds. On the Illness Scale, the former individuals are considered not as ill as the latter, and this of course makes no sense. Another problem is that subjects must have a reasonable memory for how they felt, and their reports should not be distorted by tendencies to exaggerate or minimize symptoms.[18]

Even in view of these qualifications, we still think this measure is reasonable. Surely ill people on the average will report more symptoms on more days than healthy people. To control for any tendencies to complain by some of our subjects, we also administered to them a measure of depressed mood. We assumed that if we could take this into account, we would have some perspective on their tendency to make catastrophes out of any symptoms they might experience.

We next encountered the subjects one month later—Time Two—when they again completed the Illness Scale. Of the original 172 subjects, 170 (= 99%) returned at Time Two. Note that at Time Two they were reporting on illnesses and symptoms that had occurred since Time One, when their level of optimism had been ascertained. As in the Harvard Study, our interest was in the relationship between optimism at the early point in time and health at the later point.

Finally, we contacted our subjects by letter one year later at Time Three. Enclosing a stamped envelope addressed to us, we asked:

> Would you please indicate in the space below the number of times you have visited a physician since last Thanksgiving for diagnosis and/or treatment of an illness? Do not include routine checkups or visits because of an injury (like a broken leg).

Our rationale for this measure was that the worse someone's health, the more frequently he or she might visit a doctor. Admittedly, this was not an ideal measure, but we think in general that it gave us a reasonable approximation of what we wanted to know. Of the original 172 subjects, we heard back at Time Three from 146 (= 86%). Again, we wanted to see the relationship between optimism at Time One and health measured this way at Time Three.

We have freely acknowledged the flaws in our measures because they did not prevent the emergence of the same relationship between optimism and health as in the Harvard Study. Optimistic college students—when compared to their more pessimistic peers—experienced fewer days of illness in the subsequent month and made fewer doctor visits in the subsequent year. These results held even when their initial health status (Illness Scale score at Time One) was taken into account, and even when the depression score, a plausible control for complaining, was taken into account.

The magnitudes of these relationships were somewhat less than those found in the Harvard Study, perhaps because a shorter period of time was involved. Nonetheless, their strength becomes more impressive when they are recast to compare the health status of those subjects who are among the least optimistic with those who are among the most optimistic. We compared the 25% of subjects who had the highest scores on the ASQ (the most pessimistic) with the 25% of subjects who had the lowest scores (the most optimistic). Table 2–3 gives the average number of days ill for subjects in these groups, as well as the average number of doctor visits. There is more than a two-to-one difference in the first case and more than a three-to-one difference in the second. Again, we have reason to take even these modest statistical relations seriously.

Of the subjects describing illnesses at Times One and Two, 95% described colds, sore throats, or flus. The remaining subjects reported illnesses like pneumonia, an ear infection, venereal disease, or mononucleosis. In other words, all of the illnesses were infectious. Although subjects at Time Three were not asked to describe the illnesses

TABLE 2–3. *Optimistic and Pessimistic Individuals (Common Cold Study)*

Group	Days Ill in Following Month	Doctor Visits in Following Year
pessimists (25% of sample)	8.56	3.56
optimists (25% of sample)	3.70	.95

that brought them to a physician, some small number of them did so. Every illness was infectious.

These results tell us something that the Harvard Study did not— the sort of illness to which pessimism might specifically relate. We must be cautious in expecting highly specific relationships between a psychological state and a particular health problem. Still, this finding hints at a possible path between optimism and health, one that involves the body's response to infection.

This study is not ideal. As in the Harvard Study of Adult Development, the research subjects did not constitute a cross section of the population. College students on the average are healthier, more intelligent, and more privileged than people in general. The common cold is not in the same league as cancer and heart disease, and perhaps college students—who live in close proximity to one another—are particularly at risk for colds. However, with the converging results, we began to have more confidence in the link between optimism and good health.

Two Replications of the Link between Optimism and Health

Two additional studies increased this confidence. In the first,[19] we asked 83 summer school students at the University of Michigan to complete the Attributional Style Questionnaire and to respond to the question: Are you ill right now?—definitely no—maybe—definitely yes. Subjects then kept track in a diary of any illnesses they experienced during the next three weeks. Of the 83 original subjects, 72 (= 87%) returned the diaries to us. We scored their health status as we had scored the Illness Scale in the previous study: the number of different days on which the subject experienced at least one symptom. The more optimistic the individual, the fewer days of illness he or she reported, even when answers to the "Are you ill right now?" question were taken into account statistically. Again, the magnitude of this relationship was moderate, and again, 95% of the reported symptoms seemed to suggest colds or the flu.

The second study was in some respects not so impressive as the others thus far described, because it was not longitudinal. We did not measure optimism at one point in time and health status at a later point in time. Instead, we measured both simultaneously, in what is termed a cross-sectional research design. Such designs tell us nothing about the direction of effects; the possibility that optimism leads to health is not distinguishable from the possibility that health leads to optimism. But when combined with the previous studies, this particular investigation broadens the support for our contention that at least there is a link.

Research participants in this second study were 90 middle-aged adults who as children had participated in an investigation of the effects of different styles of parental discipline.[20] Years later, in 1988, these individuals were recontacted for further study by psychologists David McClelland and Joel Weinberger of Boston University. The subjects completed a host of questionnaires and other personality measures.

Relevant to our purposes, they also wrote an essay of about 300 words in response to the following instructions:

> Please describe the worst thing that happened to you in the past year. Tell (1) when it occurred, (2) if another person was involved and who it was, (3) the gist of any conversation, and (4) what happened at the end. The other person can be anyone. The event has to be of major importance to you. Please use at least 300 words in your description.

We used the CAVE procedure described in Chapter 1 to score explanatory style from each person's essay; as in the Harvard Study, this yielded a single score for each research subject reflecting his or her habitual level of optimism versus pessimism.

Health in this study was assessed with a questionnaire that asked respondents to report on their current health status. As it turned out, optimists were healthier than pessimists, and the magnitude of this relationship was comparable to those found in our other investigations.

A Study of Optimism and Survival with Cancer

Two more confirming studies have been conducted by other researchers. Scientists are justifiably impressed by successful replications, particularly those undertaken by different research groups. We are encouraged that the link between optimistic explanatory style and good health does not depend on whatever peculiarities we might inadvertently bring to research testing this hypothesis.

In the first replication, Sandra Levy and colleagues at the University of Pittsburgh School of Medicine studied 36 middle-aged women with recurrent breast cancer.[21] Their interest was in the factors that predicted how long the women lived following the initial diagnosis of cancer. In particular, they looked at the role played by psychological factors, including optimistic explanatory style.

When the subjects initially entered the study, they were given an extensive interview that covered various topics. These interviews were then transcribed, and the CAVE procedure was used to identify, extract, and rate as optimistic or pessimistic the causal explanations of the subjects. The researchers also ascertained other factors thought to affect a woman's survival, like the extent of her cancer. And of course physicians proceeded with the appropriate treatments.

Levy and her colleagues followed the subjects for four years. Of the 36 women originally participating in this research, 24 died during this time; survival time among this group ranged from little more than 100 days to almost 1300 days (that is, 3.6 years). A number of the measures proved successful in predicting the survival time of these women, including optimism. As we would expect, the more optimistic a woman had been during the initial interview, the longer she survived.

Optimism was *not* the strongest predictor of survival time; instead, biological factors like the number of initial cancer sites were most critical. Further, the magnitude of the relationship between optimism and health (i.e., survival) was less robust than the other relationships we have described in this chapter. Levy and her colleagues exercised appropriate caution and called their results a trend. Finally, the small sample size constrained the number of possible "third variables" that could be taken into account and ruled out.

Even with limitations, these results add to the evidence for a link between optimism and physical well-being. This particular sample is not an obvious one in which to look for the effects of psychological states on health, because all of the research subjects began the study already ill—indeed, quite ill. The *onset* of illness and the *course* of illness may well have different causes. When illness has progressed far enough along, psychological factors may play a decreasing role.

A Study of Optimism and Immune System Competence

The final study was conducted by Leslie Kamen and colleagues at the University of Pennsylvania.[22] Their interest centered on the relationship between optimistic explanatory style and yet one more indicator of physical well-being: the competence of the immune system, which reflects the ability of one's body to fight off an invasion by foreign material (Chapter 5).

Like all the criteria of "health" used in optimism research, this too is far from foolproof. There are many indices of immune system competence that can be calculated from a blood sample, and spirited debate occurs among immunologists about their relative merits. Immune competence however calculated does not bear a one-to-one relationship to health and longevity; the researcher's need to rely on measures that in general are reasonable ones is again apparent.

Kamen and her colleagues conducted interviews with 47 mostly healthy adults between the ages of 62 and 87, focusing on major life events, problems, hassles, and worries. They encouraged their subjects to be mindful, and the subjects offered many causal explanations. These were scored for their level of optimism with the CAVE procedure.

A blood sample from each of the subjects, drawn at about the time the CAVE interviews were conducted, was analyzed to yield an overall estimate of immunocompetence: specifically, the ratio between T4 ("helper") cells and T8 ("suppressor") cells. The "helper" and "suppressor" labels reflect the roles that these cells play in turning on and off the body's fight against infection. So, a high ratio means a robust immune system, with relatively more helper cells and relatively fewer suppressor cells; a low ratio means a weak immune system, with relatively fewer helper cells and relatively more suppressor cells.[23]

Optimism was associated with the T4/T8 ratio, i.e., with the competence of one's immune system, to a moderate degree. Although this study used a cross-sectional design, which leaves unclear the direction of the relationship they documented, the researchers did try to rule out some likely third variables. First, an overall estimate of current health status was arrived at by two examining physicians. Someone currently ill of necessity has an immune system under attack, thus giving a misleading T4/T8 ratio. Second, each subject's level of depressed mood was estimated by a questionnaire he or she completed.[24] Research suggests that depression affects immunocompetence, again potentially biasing the T4/T8 ratio.[25] The relationship between optimism and immune system competence continued to hold even when these two measures—current health status and depressed mood—were controlled statistically.

Conclusions

The studies described in this chapter all point to the same conclusion: optimistic thinking is associated with good health, and pessimistic thinking is associated with poor health. These investigations ascertained health status in widely different ways: by physical examination; by reports of symptoms; by visits to physicians; by survival times following a cancer diagnosis; and by T4/T8 ratios reflecting immunocompetence.

This work leaves unanswered several important questions. First, we are not sure if optimism and pessimism affect the onset of illness, its course once it begins, or both. Different processes may be implicated depending on the answer to this question. And different sorts of psychological interventions may be needed depending on the answer.

Second, we do not know if the relationship between optimism and health is specific to a particular type of illness. We saw in the studies of college students that colds and the flu seem to be under the influence of pessimism, but this does not mean that other illnesses are not. Similarly, the study by Sandra Levy on survival time of patients with breast cancer shows that the course of cancer is influenced by optimism or pessimism, but again this does not mean that other illnesses are not. In the Harvard Study of Adult Development, illness was explicitly studied in nonspecific terms. The men in this study suffered from a variety of illnesses. So, we suspect a nonspecific link, but we are not entirely sure. There could be one primary health problem associated with pessimism, from which the other illnesses stem.

Third, we do not know the criterion of illness most responsive to optimism. Nor do we know the criterion that is least responsive. At least one study dramatically failed to replicate the link between optimistic explanatory style and good health. Melanie Burns and Martin Seligman at the University of Pennsylvania administered the ASQ to a group of college students, who were then given an oral thermometer and asked to keep track of their temperature for some period of time.[26] The logic here was sound. People who are ill may well run a temperature, which means that thermometers can provide an "objective" index of their physical well-being, one that does not rely on self-report and all the potential distortions thereby introduced. Healthy people should not run temperatures.

However, no association was found between explanatory style and temperature of the research subjects. Two problems become evident—after the fact. For one thing, a woman's temperature regularly rises and falls, depending on where in her menstrual cycle she happens to be. This introduces an unknown level of "noise" into the study's data, because the menstrual cycles of the female research subjects were not ascertained.

For another thing, an elevated temperature is a particularly ambiguous criterion for poor health. Yes, it shows that someone is ill. But a temperature is also a sign that a body is fighting off an infection. *Not* to have an elevated temperature during certain illnesses is a bad sign, a mark of particularly poor health. It is only when temperatures are elevated for a prolonged period of time that we have cause for alarm, and the study by Burns and Seligman did not measure temperature in so fine-grained a fashion.

Fourth, we do not understand how men and women might differ with respect to optimism and its relationship to good health. We mentioned earlier in the chapter the well-established finding in epidemiology that women have more illnesses but men die at a younger age. Stated another way, the illnesses of women are not as likely to be fatal as the illnesses of men. What if anything does optimism versus pessimism have to do with this pattern of sex differences in health?

At least on the face of it, we would think that optimism is not able to explain *both* findings. Perhaps it can explain neither. If there is a sex difference in optimism, either women are more optimistic than men, or vice versa. The sex that is more optimistic—according to the evidence we have been presenting—should have fewer illnesses *and* should live longer. Whichever is more pessimistic should have more illnesses *and* a shorter life. At the present time, we cannot even say whether men and women differ with respect to their optimism. There is no definitive evidence from our research that men and women differ in their explanatory styles, which may mean that optimism and pessimism have nothing to do with sex differences in morbidity and mortality.

We raise these unanswered questions for several reasons. One reason is simply to be honest about the state of our knowledge. We should not overstate what we know about optimism and health. The association between thinking "good" and feeling "well" seems to be pretty well-established, but we need to do a great deal more work in order to make sense of it.

Our results, however tantalizing, are merely descriptive. They do not tell us *how* optimism translates itself into good health and pessimism into poor health. So, our current research goal is to map out the biological, emotional, behavioral, and interpersonal pathways between these psychological states and physical well-being. Given the complexity of optimism as we have defined it, we expect the find these crosscutting and mutually influencing each other.

Are We Blaming the Victims of Illness?

An important issue has not yet been addressed: whether explaining illness in terms of psychological states constitutes blaming ill people for having their diseases. We know of a doctoral dissertation in progress on psychological factors that predict survival time among those who contract AIDS. This is an important and interesting topic. As it stands, AIDS has no cure. Some and maybe all who have AIDS eventually will die. On the other hand, the amount of time that people survive once they receive this diagnosis can vary greatly, from a matter of weeks to several years. The personal testimony of long-time survivors of AIDS suggests that psychological factors may be part of what makes the difference in this survival time.[27]

Isolated case studies are at best suggestive, so the idea of systematically studying psychological factors in relation to survival time is a good scientific strategy. This will tell us whether to give attention to psychological factors in the treatment of AIDS.

The dissertation author described her research to a professor whose field of expertise was AIDS. Rather than being curious or excited or simply unimpressed, he was angry. He said, "How dare you add to the misery of people who have AIDS? Isn't it enough that they are dying—do you also have to blame them for when they die?"

His reaction stemmed from his unstated but clear assumption that the *real* factors dictating survival time are biological in nature. He equated psychological explanation with moral blame. To say that a psychological variable is relevant to something that is not healthy or good is only to say that the variable makes it possible to predict who is more versus less likely to be ailing. To go one step further and say that such people are to blame for this relationship makes no more sense than to blame people who drown for the fact that their lungs didn't work too well when filled with water.

People do not freely choose their psychological operating principles any more than they choose how their lungs function. Both are in the realm of science, and hence both entail causes and effects, not free will and all of its metaphysical baggage—like sin and blame. The professor somehow interpreted psychological variables as "freely chosen" habits or beliefs that people can change at will, like clothes or the color of their fingernails. It is not that simple.

He is not alone in confusing psychological causation with moral evaluation. We see frequent warnings not to blame the victim of a disease, saddling him or her with guilt about being ill. There is enough going on when one is ill. Second-guessing one's past life is hardly the appropriate burden to add.

Along these lines, Susan Sontag has analyzed our tendencies to think about illness in terms of metaphors, appropriating notions from different domains and applying them to various illnesses.[28] Diseases that are difficult to control, lingering, and ultimately fatal in particular demand attempts to explain them, and metaphors follow. Often the metaphors are chosen from the moral domain. The problem with metaphors is that they are wrong. Indeed, it is the nature of a metaphor to be wrong.

Sontag cites tuberculosis in earlier centuries and cancer in the twentieth century as diseases explained in moral terms. AIDS has already inspired its own set of moral metaphors. People with these diseases are often seen as being responsible for them. Tuberculosis was historically linked to passion; cancer has been linked to repression; AIDS is linked to licentiousness. Thus, victims of these diseases are seen to have somehow brought about their own plight.

So we may blame victims for these diseases, and victims may blame themselves.[29] Indeed, Sontag suggests that some romantically inclined youths of the 1800s wished for tuberculosis, as proof of their sensitive nature. Needless to say, this sort of ascription of responsibility is unhelpful. It stigmatizes the individual and precludes efforts to prevent and treat illness.

Sontag is not at all interested in the possibility that psychological states contribute to illness, and she does not distinguish between psychological influences and sins. Hers is a moral argument and not a scientific one.[30] If people—including some professionals—insist on equating these, it is unfortunate. But many studies do show an influence. Part of the task of health psychologists is to spread the word not only about their results but also about the most reasonable way to look at them.

At the other extreme, it is just as irresponsible to imply that *only* psychological factors contribute to illness and death, or that people are infinitely free to choose their thoughts and beliefs. Sometimes psychological influences on health and illness are obvious and important. Sometimes they are nonexistent. It doesn't matter whether someone is an optimist or a pessimist, morally bankrupt or a saint; if she is standing in front of a speeding car she will die. Highly contagious diseases are going to spread regardless of mental outlook, and advanced illnesses will inevitably take their toll. Wishing and hoping are not going to vitiate the ultimate fact of death, extravagant claims to the contrary.[31]

We have argued strongly that psychological factors should be considered in explanations of physical well-being, and we push against a tradition that accords them no role. But we refrain from crossing sensible boundaries to say that only psychological factors matter.[32]

Where does this leave us? We are not saying that we should leave the victim alone. Smoking and drinking are "bad" habits in the sense that they have negative effects. Pessimism is a "bad" habit as well, for precisely the same reason. Certainly aggressive steps should be taken to encourage people to change their bad habits. But these steps do not entail blaming them in a moral sense for the habits they have developed, even when psychological factors are 100% implicated. Here we join ranks with those who counsel against saddling ill people with extra baggage.

One of the truisms in psychotherapy is that fixing blame and finding solutions are very different matters. Clients sometimes do not grasp the distinction, because there is something satisfying about blaming problems on one's spouse, or one's business partners, or the intolerance of the world, or government policies. Many times blame is correctly allocated. But blame is the business of God or the police department, whereas solutions are the business of the therapist. The client must learn to separate the past from the future.[33] There are no shortcuts, no sudden insights, no pain-free solutions.

3

Positive Thoughts
and Good Health

Too much of a good thing
is wonderful.

— *Mae West*

An optimistic style of explaining
events has been linked to good health; a pessimistic one to poor
health. The studies described in Chapter 2 strengthen our belief that
psychological states can affect physical well-being. We will now focus
on other studies that further suggest an association of positive
thoughts with good health. These constitute a rapidly developing
body of work to which we cannot do full justice in the present chapter, but we will describe a few lines of inquiry that converge with our
own. The recent successful attempts to link psychological states and
health have given rise to some discord, and we conclude by comment-
ing on this.

Lines of Related Research

We start here with work quite similar to our own, then move to somewhat different topics.

Dispositional optimism   Psychologists Michael Scheier and Charles
Carver have for several years investigated the relationship to physical

health of a personality characteristic they call dispositional optimism.[1] Their work, of all that to be discussed, bears the closest resemblance to our own.

They define dispositional optimism as one's general expectation that the future holds good outcomes. It is presumably a general and stable characteristic that people have to varying extents. Scheier and Carver measure dispositional optimism with a questionnaire called the Life Orientation Test. This measure is called the LOT for short. The humor of the acronym may be intentional: the test measures people's expectations about their "lot" in life. Respondents are shown statements like the following:

• In uncertain times, I usually expect the best.
• If something can go wrong, it will.

Obviously, the first example epitomizes optimism; the second, pessimism.

Someone responding to the LOT chooses numbers from 1 to 5 that indicate the degree to which he or she agrees with each statement. High scores indicate optimism, and low scores indicate pessimism. Using this questionnaire, Scheier and Carver have done a series of studies that link optimism to good health and pessimism to poor health. For instance, college students who were pessimists reported more somatic symptoms at a given point in time and developed more symptoms at a later point than did those who were optimists, even when initial levels of symptoms were controlled statistically.[2] In another study, this one of men who underwent coronary artery bypass surgery, optimism was related not only to the making of active plans and the setting of goals for recovery but additionally to better recovery six months later.[3] The optimistic men were more likely to have returned to work and to have resumed recreational, social, and sexual activities. They were also more likely to be exercising vigorously.

Hardiness Another personality characteristic linked to physical well-being that overlaps considerably with our notion of optimism versus pessimism is hardiness. The focus of research by Suzanne Kobasa, hardiness is conceived as varying from individual to individual.[4] According to Kobasa, people who are more hardy approach the world with curiosity, finding meaning and interest at every turn. Hardy individuals can accommodate change in their life and are able to recast stressful events as challenges. They take an optimistic perspective whenever possible. In contrast, those who are less hardy find the world either boring or overwhelming. They are passive and pessimistic.

Hardiness spans three entwined dimensions: commitment, control, and challenge.[5] Commitment refers to someone's involvement in personal projects and goals. Someone scoring high on commitment is personally engaged; someone scoring low is merely going through the motions. Control entails a belief that important outcomes can be controlled and solutions to the problems of life can be devised. Someone high in control actively confronts her surrounding world; someone low is fatalistic, expecting luck or fate to prevail. Finally, challenge refers to the way that stressful events are construed. These can be looked at as opportunities for personal growth, or as threats to esteem and security.

Hardiness is measured with a questionnaire that presents respondents with various questions reflecting its three components. To the degree that they agree with these statements, they are considered hardy. Studies show that hardiness measured this way predicts which people are less likely to fall ill when they experience stress. For instance, one study compared 100 working adults with numerous complaints of illness with 100 other working adults who had few complaints.[6] Although each group had experienced the same number of stressful events, the second group proved to be hardier than the first. A second study found the same results among 157 attorneys in general practice.[7] Yet another study followed executives over time, again finding that hardiness conferred on them immunity against illness.[8]

Kobasa's research on hardiness has been criticized for the way she goes about measuring the notion. Critics observe that it is difficult to identify the active force among the three psychological dimensions that her measure spans, because the questionnaire lumps them all together. Does this difficulty call into question her findings?

All measures are flawed, and the best a researcher can do is look for convergence of results across studies using different measures. And results here do point to the same conclusion—whether the researchers have measured explanatory style, dispositional optimism, or hardiness. Presumably, the flaws of different lines of research are offsetting.

Self-efficacy   Another concept related to optimism and pessimism as we construe them is self-efficacy, introduced by psychologist Albert Bandura.[9] Self-efficacy is a person's belief that he can perform a particular behavior that will produce a particular outcome. The idea emerged from Bandura's studies of behavior modification—how to use reward and punishment to help people change in beneficial ways (Chapter 7). In its original version, the theory behind behavior modification emphasized the environment: the manipulation of rewards and punishments to get someone to behave in a certain way or to refrain from doing so.

As Bandura investigated how people changed their behavior (or did not) in response to environmental manipulations, he realized that while outside factors were important, there were other influences on behavior change. It was all well and good to arrange situations so that a particular reward or punishment followed a particular response, but this would have no effect on whether a person performed the behavior in question unless the person believed that he was capable of doing so.

In a number of studies, Bandura demonstrated that people's belief in their own ability to perform a particular behavior (efficacy) strongly predicted whether or not they would perform it. This belief proves to be a more potent influence on future behavior than an individual's past behavior. There are few generalizations in psychology, but one of the best established is that past behavior predicts future behavior; there is considerable inertia in thinking and feeling and acting. Self-efficacy is an exception to this generalization and thus worthy of note.

What is the relevance of self-efficacy to health? Anne O'Leary did an extensive literature review:

> The evidence taken as a whole is consistent in showing that people's perceptions of their efficacy are related to different forms of health behavior. In the realm of substance abuse, perceived self-regulatory efficacy is a reliable predictor of who will relapse and the circumstances of each person's first slip. Strong percepts of efficacy to manage pain increase pain tolerance. . . . [Perceived efficacy with regard to] . . . eating and weight predicts who will succeed in overcoming eating disorders. Recovery from the severe trauma of myocardial infarction is tremendously facilitated by the enhancement of the patients' and their spouses' judgments of their physical and cardiac capabilities. And self-efficacy to affect one's own health increases adherence to medical regimens. . . . While specific procedures may differ for different domains, the general strategy of assessing and enhancing self-percepts of efficacy to affect health . . . has substantial general utility.[10]

Stripped of jargon, O'Leary's statement says that people behave in healthful ways to the degree that they believe they can enact specific behaviors that are pertinent (or refrain from them). Indeed, self-efficacy may be one of the critical factors underlying people's adherence to diets and other health-promoting activities.[11]

That self-efficacy may have a direct effect on health is shown in recent studies by Bandura and his colleagues of how people's physiological responses to stress are influenced by their levels of self-efficacy with respect to coping responses. The more people believe they can cope with stress, the less the toll that stress takes on their bodies.[12] Other related studies suggest that people with enhanced self-efficacy have more robust immune systems.[13]

In the next chapter, we discuss the origins of optimistic explanatory style, and our conclusions dovetail with Bandura's hypotheses about the determinants of self-efficacy.[14] According to Bandura, people arrive at their beliefs concerning their own efficacy—or lack thereof—by attending to four sources of information.

First is the individual's history of actual successes and failures. The more success a person experiences, the more likely he is to believe that future success is within his grasp, and he thus becomes increasingly efficacious in this particular domain. It is critical that the individual perceive success as something that follows from his own actions. Goodies handed out like Halloween candy constitute no kind of success at all, at least in terms of strengthening self-efficacy. There is an interesting implication here: permissiveness can undercut efficacy, if it encourages the person to think less of his own competence.

The second way that a person's self-efficacy is encouraged (or thwarted) is by watching other people succeed (or fail). Bandura is well known to students of psychology for introducing the idea of modeling; he proposed that a great deal of what people learn to do appears not gradually through trial and error but rather all at once following the observation of what other people—called models—are doing. So, people come to believe that they can have desired effects on the world by seeing that others do. And just as easily, they can come to believe in their own lack of self-efficacy by watching others fail.

A qualification is needed, however. Someone is affected by models to the degree that the models appear similar to the person, are likable, and/or meet with reward for whatever they are doing (even if it is failing). We suspect that modeling plays a large role in the contagion of optimism and pessimism, a phenomenon we discuss in Chapter 6.

Another determinant of self-efficacy is exhortation or persuasion. This may be explicit, as in a pep talk by a coach: "You can do it."

Or it may be subtle, overlapping with the process of modeling. Optimistic or pessimistic beliefs may be acquired not only through direct experience but also by listening to others who urge positive or negative outlooks upon us. However, we strongly doubt that any single communication will be effective in turning a pessimist into an optimist. Optimism and pessimism are much more global concepts than are particular beliefs about self-efficacy, which are specific to given actions. They thus resist our simple attempts to change them to a much greater degree. We will discuss how optimism and pessimism change in Chapter 7.

The fourth determinant of self-efficacy is the physiological feedback that accompanies our actions. Activity that is effortless leads to a belief in self-efficacy. In contrast, people may conclude that they are not meeting the demands of a task when their bodies are tired, or tense, or breathless, or sweaty. They doubt their own ability in light of this feedback and diminish (accordingly) their sense of self-efficacy. Needless to say, this doubt can be fallacious—instilled by a society that does not approve of perspiration.

The practical implication is that people need to rethink what it means to be in control of one's life. The prototype of a person high in self-efficacy should not be someone cool, calm, and collected but someone active, excited, vigorous, and even sweaty. Remember the point in Chapter 1 that optimism is beneficial precisely because it leads someone to activity; activity further strengthens the sense of self-efficacy.

Social support   Other people are good for our health. We hesitate not at all in making this assertion, because it has ample support in the research literature.[15] For instance, a variety of problems are more common among those who are isolated from others than among those not at the fringes of social life. Their immune systems are less competent. They suffer more from emotional disorders. Their life expectancy is reduced by every friend or family member they do not have. They even experience more automobile "accidents" than people who have friends and family![16] Many of these generalizations hold even when these individuals make more money or cultivate fewer bad habits (e.g., smoking or drinking) than their more socially enmeshed counterparts.

Just how is it that other people work their magic upon our well-being? Psychologists attack this question by asking just what it is that other people do for us, using the term "social support" to capture the various benefits that people can provide to one another.[17] Among the benefits that can be specified are:

- emotional reassurance
- provision of tangible resources, like money or food
- advice about tackling problems
- perspective—telling a person that how he or she sees things is all right

Needless to say, an indefinite number of influences can be classified under the heading of social support. Many are highly specific to health and its promotion. Consider attempts to quit smoking or lose weight; the presence of an encouraging friend or spouse can make all the difference in the world. And the different manifestations of support may strengthen each other, opening up doors on good health and closing those on bad health.

The crux of social support should not be misunderstood. It is not a matter of trying to "receive" as much as one can from other people while giving nothing in return. Social support reflects the degree to which people find themselves in supportive *relationships:* two-way streets. Indeed, a study has found that people who do regular volunteer work show a dramatic increase in life expectancy over those who perform no such services for others.[18] The study followed several thousand individuals over a ten-year period. Among the men in the study, those who did no volunteer work were two and a half times as likely to die during this period than were those who did volunteer work at least once a week.[19] Apparently critical in determining who most benefits from volunteer work is the person's freedom of choice in deciding just what type of activity will be pursued, from answering a telephone hotline to delivering meals to the housebound.

One of the most interesting lines of research on influence of others on health is James Pennebaker's investigations of "confession" and physical well-being. In one study, he contacted the spouses of individuals who had died by suicide or accident one year after their death.[20] Subjects were asked to indicate how they had responded to the death of their mate as well as enumerate the health problems they had encountered during the last year. The results were striking:

- The more frequently that subjects discussed their spouse's death with other people, the fewer health problems they experienced.

- The more they ruminated about the death, the more health problems they had.
- To the degree that they discussed the death with others, they ruminated less.

Further studies by Pennebaker and his colleagues showed that confiding in other people has particular physiological effects, suggesting that the apparent link between confiding and good health reflects at least in part a biological pathway.[21] The point we would like to emphasize about this fascinating work is that confiding is inherently a social endeavor. The expression of one's sins and secrets and hopes and fears to others may bring relief which translates itself into good health.

Perhaps this point is relevant to the finding that those who attend church are in better health than those who do not; they also live longer.[22] The linkage holds regardless of the type of church in question, so it is probably not the content of the beliefs per se that makes a difference but rather the fact of holding them—and doing so in the context of a group. To feel oneself part of some larger entity is apparently conducive to health. This benefit may be at least partly behind the rapid growth in recent years of support groups for people confronting all sorts of difficulties in life: substance abuse, divorce, assault, and so on.

We will explain in Chapter 6 how optimistic people are precisely those who are socially enmeshed. Pessimists are socially estranged, alienated and alienating. They do not have the same sort of supportive friendships that optimists do.[23]

Stress   One of the topics most frequently investigated by psychologists during the 1980s was stress. Stress itself is difficult to define, sometimes referring to external events that make demands on an individual and sometimes to the response of the individual to these demands. Regardless, studies of stress have led investigators to appreciate further the important role that our thoughts and beliefs play in our lives.

Hans Selye introduced an influential description of the body's response to threatening events.[24] He found that regardless of the stressor, its continued presence leads to the same sequence of physiological reactions. He called this sequence the general adaptation syndrome. It proceeds from mobilization of the body's resources to resistance against stress to eventual exhaustion if the stressor is not overcome.

The general adaptation syndrome is helpful in explaining why different problems may occur together. In using bodily resources to resist one stressor, an individual is less likely to have these resources available to cope with other stressors. The course of a particular disease, for instance, may be influenced by the presence or absence of other diseases.

Stress has been linked to illness in a number of well-controlled studies.[25] Investigators Thomas Holmes and Richard Rahe created the Social Readjustment Rating Scale to gauge the *quantity* of stress a person has been experiencing.[26] In responding to this questionnaire, a research subject indicates which of 43 major life events occurred in the past year (see Table 3–1). The more an event disrupts someone's ongoing life and requires adjustment, the higher the "life change unit" score associated with the event. As the total score on this scale increases, the more likely the person is to fall ill.

It is not just major life events that create stress. Indeed, Kanner, Coyne, Schaefer, and Lazarus created a measure that parallels the Social Readjustment Rating Scale, except that it asks about hassles: small but annoying events in the course of daily life, such as losing car keys, being interrupted at dinner, making a mistake while balancing one's checkbook, or having to take care of someone else's pet.[27] As hassles accumulate, so does stress, taking a toll on physical well-being. In their sheer numbers, hassles may be even more stressful than major life events.[28]

Once the stress-illness link was established, researchers began to take a look at its nature, and they found that psychological factors were critical. Specifically, an event becomes stressful and likely to lead to illness to the degree that one thinks about it in a particular way. Consider the individual who makes catastrophes out of minor disappointments:

> I had a bad time on my date last night.
> It seems I've always had bad times on dates.
> Plus my job doesn't go much better.
> My boss frowned at me last week.
> I can't figure out how to work my computer.
> I'm not good at anything.

This woman has worked herself into a dither by her way of thinking. Suppose she had said instead about her date, "He must have been tired—that's why we didn't have a good time"?

TABLE 3–1. *Stressful Life Events*

Event	"Life change unit" score
1. death of spouse	100
2. divorce	73
3. marital separation	65
4. jail term	63
5. death of a close family member	63
6. major personal injury or illness	53
7. marriage	50
8. being fired at work	47
9. marital reconciliation	45
10. retirement	45
11. major change in health of family member	44
12. pregnancy	40
13. sexual difficulties	39
14. gaining a new family member	39
15. major business readjustment	39
16. major change in financial state	38
17. death of close friend	37
18. changing to a different line of work	36
19. major change in number of arguments with spouse	35
20. taking out a mortgage or loan for a major purchase	31
21. foreclosure on a mortgage or loan	30
22. major change in responsibilities at work	29
23. son or daughter leaving home	29
24. trouble with in-laws	29
25. outstanding personal achievement	28
26. spouse begins or ceases work outside the home	26
27. beginning or ending school	26
28. major change in living conditions	25
29. revision of personal habits	24
30. trouble with boss	23
31. major change in working hours or conditions	20
32. change in residence	20
33. changing to a new school	20
34. major change in usual type and/or amount of recreation	19

TABLE 3–1. *Stressful Life Events* (continued)

35. major change in church activities	19
36. major change in social activities	18
37. taking out a mortgage or loan for a minor purchase	17
38. major change in sleeping habits	16
39. major change in number of family get-togethers	15
40. major change in eating habits	15
41. vacation	13
42. Christmas	12
43. minor violations of the law	11

SOURCE: Reprinted with permission from *Journal of Psychosomatic Research, 11,* T. H. Holmes and R. H. Rahe, "The Social Readjustment Rating Scale," Copyright © 1967, Pergamon Press plc.

Researchers have discovered a number of ways of thinking that magnify the stressful effects of events. The more that one regards events as unpredictable and uncontrollable, the more stressful they are. Conflict about events can also cause stress. And when one blames oneself for bad events but feels powerless to change them, they too are particularly stressful. In some cases, these beliefs reflect the reality of the situation; in other cases, they go beyond the facts of the matter and create unnecessary stress for the person. One way to describe the thrust of these findings is to say that a pessimistic view of life events makes them more stressful and thus more likely to produce illness.[29] Conversely, an upbeat way of thinking may serve as a buffer against the health-threatening effects of stress.

Coping One of the best known investigators of the ways in which people cope with stress is Richard Lazarus.[30] He takes a thoroughly cognitive approach, arguing that the stressfulness of a particular situation depends on how someone appraises it and his ability to meet its demands.

Lazarus proposes that two types of appraisal are important. The first, primary appraisal, refers to the individual's interpretation of what is at stake. Suppose a person receives a traffic ticket for speeding in a residential area. No one likes to get a ticket, of course, but his emotional reaction will vary greatly depending on whether he is required to go to court, how much he might be fined, whether his driving record is good or bad, and whether his car insurance rates might be raised. What seems to be the same event—being given a traffic ticket—takes on wholly different forms depending on how its consequences are appraised.

In secondary appraisal, the person assesses the resources she has available to cope with a stressful event. She perceives some negative situations as easily resolved: by waiting them out, by talking to someone in charge, by regarding them as a joke and/or a good lesson. Distress following such events is minimal. Other negative occurrences are seen as not so easy to cope with, and considerable distress follows.

Lazarus further distinguishes between coping strategies that are problem-focused and those that are emotion-focused. In problem-focused coping, one tries to change the world to remove the source of stress. A broken television set usually demands problem-focused coping. In emotion-focused coping, one tries to change how one is feeling about an event. A broken heart usually demands emotion-focused coping.

> . . . give us grace to accept with serenity the things that cannot be changed, courage to change the things which should be changed, and the wisdom to distinguish the one from the other.
> —*Reinhold Niebuhr (1892–1971)*

Let us echo Lazarus's caution that there is no best coping strategy for all circumstances. The most effective coping depends on the person and on the particular stressor she faces. Regardless, the optimistic person attempts to cope in some way with stressful events, whereas the pessimist is at a loss. In subsequent chapters, we will discuss several studies that document this link between optimism and active coping.

Inhibited power motivation   Another body of work implicating the role of psychological factors in susceptibility to poor health has resulted from psychologist David McClelland's investigation of power motivation: someone's need to have an impact on other people. Some people have a strong need for power; others, a weak one. Power motivation per se has no simple effect on health. Instead, McClelland found that people with a high need for power who constantly inhibit its expression end up at risk.

It is worth exploring some of the details of McClelland's work. One way to measure an individual's level of power motivation is by giving him projective tests. The research subject is shown an ambiguous picture—one that is objectively fuzzy and able to be seen in various ways—and asked to describe what is going on in the picture. McClelland favors a projective test known as the Thematic Apperception Test (TAT), a series of pictures that have characters in them, although it is not quite clear what they are doing. A subject is asked to tell a story with a beginning, middle, and end, and then the researcher codes the story for mention of various themes that indicate particular needs. In the case of power motivation, he or she looks for characters having an impact on one another. The more themes per story, the higher the subject scores on this motive.

The inhibition of power motivation is scored very straightforwardly, by looking for negations of these themes: i.e., if the word "not" appears in the descriptions. The more negations, the more inhibited the storyteller is with respect to power motivation. The Ten Commandments, for instance, which abound with "thou shalt nots" vis-à-vis other people, would receive a high score on this scoring system.

Although the TAT and other projective tests can be difficult to score, McClelland has successfully linked inhibited power motivation as scored from the TAT to physical well-being.[31] Among the striking findings he noted was the involvement of this characteristic—and several other motive patterns—in alcoholism, diabetes, high blood pressure, and respiratory infections. Stated another way, people who want to have an impact on others but hold this need in check are not as healthy as those who either do not possess a strong need for power *or* who give expression to this need. Other studies suggest that inhibited power and other motives are linked to depressed immune functioning in the wake of stress. McClelland urges a cautious view of these findings, noting that they can be complex. At the same time, they appear to support the linkage of psychological states with health.

Type A behavior pattern   One of the most familiar constellations of psychological characteristics related to health is the Type A coronary-prone behavior pattern. There is an apocryphal story about the first hint that certain ways of behaving were linked specifically to heart disease. A coronary specialist always sent the chairs from his office to the same upholsterer when the seats became worn. The upholsterer, who had repaired and returned the chairs several times, remarked that he never had any trouble knowing which office these chairs came from. The seats were always worn in the same unusual way—all of them were worn out at the very front, as if the people sitting in them were always perched on the edge.

That of course is the point: those at risk for heart disease behave in characteristic ways, and we would expect that if ever there were people who always sat on the edge of their seats it would be this group. Researchers began to take a close look at this hypothesis, and a clear pattern soon emerged.[32]

The behavior of those at risk for heart disease could be subsumed under three general categories. These people were time-urgent, always watching clocks, always hurrying off to appointments. They were hostile, particularly in the face of demands made on them. ("What's it to you buddy? What do you mean my car is standing on your foot?") And finally, they were competitive.

The Type A constellation is assessed either by interview or by a questionnaire. In either case, questions tap the degree to which the subjects show the cardinal features. A particularly high scoring individual is a Type A; a particularly low scoring one, a Type B. Some are intermediate, obviously. Researchers usually compare the two groups at the extremes.

Being a Type A is a mixed blessing. Researchers have become intrigued by the concept and have explored not only its possible link to heart disease but also its relationship to other aspects of functioning in daily life. Type A individuals indeed are go-getters and achievers.[33] As students, they get better grades than sheer ability might suggest; they hold more class offices; they do better in athletics. As workers, they work hard and well. They make lots of money. They also are at risk for illness and death before their time.[34]

More recent research suggests that the critical ingredient in the Type A pattern—with respect to heart disease—is hostility.[35] But the link between hostility and heart disease may not be direct and physiological. It could well be interpersonal, because the hostility of the Type A may turn off other people and thereby preclude the benefits of social support that we discussed earlier.[36] It might also reflect demoralization, because the Type A individual creates a world for herself in which frustrations abound, eventually to take their toll on her mood. As we will describe in Chapter 5, depression has itself been linked to poor health.

An ironic aspect of research on the Type A pattern is that it sometimes proves difficult to slow down Type A individuals long enough for them to complete the interviews or questionnaires via which they are to be assessed. They are too impatient to answer questions, particularly in studies that follow the same people over time. Needless to say, such studies are exactly the way to learn just how and why Type As are sometimes at risk for poor health.

What is the relationship between optimism and the Type A pattern? Type As show an intense drive to succeed and to control their environments.[37] Sometimes they succeed, but what happens when control proves elusive? Studies have been conducted in which laboratory tasks for Type A subjects were arranged so that they could not master them.[38] At first, the Type A individual makes a heroic effort to perform the task. When this fails, she becomes passive and despondent.

One way to look at these results is to propose that type A individuals are prone to pessimism when roadblocks are placed in their way that they cannot readily surmount by sheer brute force. Other lines of evidence confirm this hypothesis. Brunson and Matthews found that when failure is imposed on a Type A individual, she shows dysfunctional strategies of solving problems, more so than a Type B individual.[39] For instance, a Type A person might perseverate in a way that is clearly proving to be fruitless. Also, a Type A, in response to failure, is apt to blame herself for the difficulties she experiences. Type Bs offer more upbeat explanations; they entertain the idea that the difficulty of a task had something to do with why they failed at it. Regardless, they approach problem solving more flexibly.

We do not know the exact relationship between Type A behavior and optimism versus pessimism as we measure it with the ASQ,[40] although we are in the process of exploring it in a study with colleagues here at the University of Michigan. Type A will not reduce to pessimism, we can be sure, nor will pessimism reduce to Type A. What is important is that these constructs overlap and that both draw our attention to how people respond to failure, how they perceive the causes of events, and how they approach the problems posed by life.

Bereavement   Can a person die of a broken heart? This is a widespread belief, and most of us have heard of a grieving spouse who followed his or her mate to death. But isolated examples do not show this to be a valid generalization. Indeed, the notion of a broken heart is dismissed in some quarters as romanticism. However, when we take a hard-headed look at the evidence, the idea that illness and death are more likely following the loss of a loved one is solidly supported.[41] We draw here on the work recently reported by Wolfgang Stroebe and Margaret Stroebe.[42]

They surveyed studies by other researchers as well as conducting their own investigation. Most of the research looks at the consequences of losing a husband or wife to death. To quote their conclusions:

> . . . the convergence of these findings is quite impressive. Whether one looks at the rate of . . . physical illness . . . or mortality, comparisons of married and widowed individuals typically find the widowed to be worse off. . . . The experience of partner loss is associated with health deterioration.[43]

Indeed, in the research by Holmes and Rahe that we described earlier, the single most stressful life event is the death of one's spouse (see Table 3–1).

Of course, not all who lose a partner suffer poor health, so we must ask who is more or less at risk for poor health while bereaved? According to Stroebe and Stroebe, several factors combine to put an individual at particular risk. If a death was unexpected—because the spouse was young or a victim of an accident or a crime—then the mourner's health will suffer more than if the death were more expected, as due to old age or a lingering illness. The unexpected death of a spouse leaves someone with "unfinished business" in the marriage that can never be resolved.

Another factor related to the extent to which a person's health suffers following bereavement is the degree that the death of the spouse seems meaningless. Compare losing a husband in war to losing one to a senseless accident. Although not everyone can find meaning in a war death, certainly this is an easier thing to do than to understand a death that is due to choking on a bite of food or being hit by a drunken driver. Sudden death is so shocking that survivors have difficulty accommodating themselves to it; "meaning" is slow to take form, if it does at all. However, if meaning can be found, then the survivor's health is protected to a degree.[44]

Yet another factor influencing the effect of bereavement on the subsequent health of the survivor is the degree of support that she garners from other people. The more people who are present and supportive, the less her health will suffer. As we have already discussed, people who have many and substantial friendships are healthier than those who do not, so this qualification may simply be a special case of the more general buffering effect that supportive contacts play.

The physician who attends to the dying person is in a unique position to offer support to the surviving family members, yet a study by Susan Tolle and colleagues suggests that support by physicians is not common.[45] They interviewed the spouses of 105 adults who died one year earlier at a hospital. Fewer than half of these individuals had spoken *at all* to the attending physician in the year that had passed. Yet many of them had questions that remained unanswered. Could the death have been prevented? Had an autopsy been performed? What transpired at the very end of the spouse's life? A sincere attempt to answer questions like these might help the mourners achieve some sense of closure on the loss they had experienced.

On the face of it, the results of this study seem outrageous, evidence for a lack of respect and concern on the part of physicians for those they serve—both living and dead. But when we described these findings to a friend, he was not surprised. His comments gave us another perspective. "Maybe the doctors are afraid of being sued if they say they are sorry." Could this be true? We know that physicians and patients are increasingly antagonistic toward one another.[46] Perhaps the findings by Tolle and her colleagues are just one more sign of the problem.

Research suggests that women adjust somewhat better than men to the loss of a spouse.[47] Two reasons come to mind. The first is that widows far outnumber widowers in our society. The loss of one's husband is thus more expected. The second is that women may be more likely than men to seek the support of others in a time of loss, thereby garnering some protective benefits.

Being widowed does not mean being at constant risk for poor health. The risk appears limited to the six months following a loss. This could mean that those who are going to succumb do so immediately, but a better interpretation is probably that by then most widows have regained their resilience. Supporting this idea is research on immune functioning following bereavement. Investigators have shown, for instance, that a griever's immune functioning is suppressed for several months following her bereavement, but then it rebounds.[48]

What is the connection between these findings on bereavement and our work on optimism and health? In the most general terms, the fact that bereavement can lead to poor health and even death is consistent with our argument that psychological factors influence people's physical well-being. More specifically, studies of bereavement show that people who are unable to achieve cognitive and emotional closure following the loss of a loved one are particularly apt to suffer in its aftermath. Stated yet another way, those most at risk for dying of a broken heart are those who cannot take an optimistic approach to that part of their life that goes on.

Common Themes

We have described nine lines of research that support the work we discussed in detail in Chapter 2 linking optimism and health. There seems little doubt that psychological states can and do influence one's physical well-being. Recent books by Ornstein and Sobel, Justice, and Locke and Colligan, among others,[49] cite hundreds of studies by researchers at the forefront of what Justice terms the "heady revolution"—the belated discovery that one's thoughts and feelings indeed affect one's mortality and morbidity.

People have tried for thousands of years to identify the influence of mind on health, as we will discuss in Chapter 8; why does the "heady revolution" seem to be succeeding now? The answer to this question is that psychologists have finally hit upon the right aspect of "mind" to look at. Here is what we mean, in terms of the common emphases in the disparate lines of work cited above:

1. It is people's manifest thoughts and beliefs that pertain most directly to their health. Previous researchers looked mainly at emotions, conflicts, and/or unconscious processes, and the yield was much more modest.
2. It is how someone thinks in particular about setbacks and disappointments that matters. Philosopher Charles Peirce wrote that the purpose of thought is to allay doubt,[50] and the current generation of psychological researchers has had the good fortune to zero in on people under circumstances where they are most likely to be mindful.
3. It is thoughts about the real world—its events, their causes, and their aftermath—that relate to well-being.
4. It is thoughts that are responsive to other people that are pertinent.
5. It is the sorts of beliefs that lead to action, that are infused with agency and efficacy, that lead to health. Those that result in passivity and demoralization do not.

Not all lines of work that psychologists are pursuing exemplify all of these emphases. Some slide into the emotional/motivational realm and others into a purely ideational one. Some more directly address "reality" than others. Nonetheless, there is convergence in the vicinity of what we have called optimism.

Attacks from the Medical Establishment

To call a series of studies a revolution can be to indulge in hyperbole, but in this case the term is literal. To revolt is to revolt against something, and we do indeed find resistance in some quarters against the ideas we are presenting. Although many doctors are wise and tolerant, we feel that the medical establishment, as it were, deserves some criticism. This establishment is not just skeptical of the possibility that minds influence bodies but also on occasion is downright obstructive.

We will support this contention by examining one particular instance, an editorial published in the highly prestigious *New England Journal of Medicine*. The apparent trigger for the editorial was two studies previously published in this journal that sought—without success—some role of psychological factors in illness.

Cassileth et al. studied several hundred cancer patients,[51] looking at a number of factors that might play a role in predicting their survival time:

- social ties and marital history
- job satisfaction
- use of drugs
- general life satisfaction
- subjective view of health
- degree of hopelessness and helplessness
- perception of the amount of adjustment required to cope with the diagnosis

We have just cited study after study showing that such factors are correlated with good health. But in this particular investigation, none of these was correlated with how long the patients survived. Instead, somatic factors—like the size of the tumor—proved more important.

Is this an exemplary study? We think not, because it falls short of satisfying several criteria we proposed earlier as necessary to investigate the role of psychological factors (pp. 23–24). The particular measures were not well described by Cassileth et al. Apparently the authors did not consider the possibility that asking patients to fill out questionnaires in the immediate aftermath of cancer diagnosis and treatment might make their answers less useful than if such measures were administered under less stressful circumstances.

Furthermore, the initial health of the patients was not taken into account when the influence of psychological factors on subsequent health was calculated. Curiously, this information was apparently available, if the size of one's tumor has something to do with the severity of cancer, but data analyses did not include psychological and somatic factors simultaneously. More generally, is it surprising that among a group of patients whose cancer had progressed to the point where the majority of them died, psychological variables were swamped? This particular group seems not to be the best place to look for psychological factors.

The second study was one that ascertained the Type A behavior pattern of 516 patients within two weeks after each had suffered an acute myocardial infarction.[52] These patients were then followed for three years, and it was found that their Type A scores showed no relationship to later heart problems, measured in various ways. Also, mortality was not related to Type A scores. Physiological factors showed the only demonstrable relationship to what ensued.

Again, this is not an exemplary study for showing that psychological factors influence health. Is there a theoretical reason for thinking that Type A behaviors should affect the *aftermath* of heart disease?[53] Did these subjects modify their behavior in light of the problems they experienced? Can a researcher validly assess Type A behaviors while a person is recovering from a heart attack? The researchers acknowledged this problem:

> It should be noted that the JAS [a Type A measure] was administered after infarction. Questions can be raised concerning the usefulness of recording such data after the cardiac event, since patients with Type A behavior may have an increased fatality rate with their infarction, resulting in a behaviorally selected population.[54]

But they focused only on the possibility of a restricted range of scores, not on the more general issue of the measure's validity.

Regardless, these two studies were cited by Marcia Angell, the deputy editor of the *New England Journal of Medicine,* in an editorial warning against psychological explanations of health and illness.[55] "The literature contains very few scientifically sound studies of the relation, if there is one, between mental state and disease," she declared,[56] ignoring the hundreds of studies that do point to such a link. Her own editorial contained only nine references, including three to popular books and one to a newspaper article.

Angell argued that the attempt to explain illness in psychological terms is more than simply wrong; it is also dangerous. It encourages the patient with an illness to blame himself if recovery is not rapid or complete.

> What about the patients who *don't* survive? Are they lacking the will to live, or perhaps self-discipline or some other personal attribute necessary to hold cancer at bay?[57]

The person with such a belief is apt to feel guilty and inadequate in the face of any illness, and this is not good, she observed.

We cannot resist asking, in light of Angell's desire to reduce everything to biology and dismiss altogether psychological factors, just why it should matter whether someone feels guilty or inadequate. Guilt is not a biological state; it is a psychological one. We also believe that it is not healthy for people to feel guilty and inadequate, precisely because these feelings can contribute to illness in their own right.

Angell concluded her editorial by branding the belief that disease reflects mental states "folklore" that we would all be better off without. Theorists and researchers involved in establishing the link between psychological states and health were quick to respond to her opinions. The *New England Journal* published a number of replies, many pointing out the voluminous research literature that Angell ignored.

In August 1985, the American Psychological Association—the largest professional organization of psychologists—passed a resolution criticizing the editorial as "inaccurate" and urging that the relevant information be made available to the larger public.[58] In a later response to the criticisms, Angell backed down from her position, to some extent,[59] but her reply strikes us as ingenuous. She argued that while she was accused of trying to suppress research, this was not her intention. (If an editorial about unproductive lines of inquiry by an editor of the best known medical journal in the world is not meant to influence what researchers do, then what is the point?) She then called the evidence about mind-body links "inconclusive," and said that people have such a strong desire to believe that mental states influence disease that they may be blinded to the actual lack of a relationship.

Debates Within Psychology

It is not the case that physicians wear black hats and psychologists white ones. There is a trend in psychology that we find as disturbing as any in medicine. We fear it will distract psychologists from making a genuine contribution to understanding and—eventually—treating illness.

In another example of the "nothing but" approach we criticized in Chapter 1, psychologists interested in health and illness have a growing tendency to acknowledge on the one hand that psychological factors influence well-being, but then on the other hand to argue that it is only a particular notion measured in a particular way that is worthy of attention.

Unstated in these arguments is that much research into health and illness requires funding from the federal government, and that the overall amount of money is severely limited. One researcher's success at earning research support necessarily depends on the failure of others to secure funding. What results is squabbling and jealousy. What is best for the larger society is lost from view.

A recent convention of psychologists included a special symposium on the influence of psychological factors on physical health. The symposium degenerated into feuding and sniping among the panel members—all of whom were solid researchers whose work we respect—about whose measures were more flawed. Some of the panel members were so unpleasant to one another that many of those in attendance walked out well before the conclusion of the presentations.

Our approach to warring factions is to take a broader look, and we find striking convergence in different lines of work. Indeed, all measures are flawed, as we noted earlier. To the degree that they yield comparable conclusions, we should be impressed. Science does not rise and fall on single findings so much as on a web of results; as they are woven together, they gather strength not found in single threads.

The Origins of Optimism

Words are more powerful than
perhaps anyone suspects, and
once deeply engraved in a child's
mind, they are not easily
eradicated.

— *May Sarton*

W e know more about the conse-
quences of optimism and pessimism than we do about their origins.
However, our purpose in this chapter is to sketch what we have so far
learned about the influences early in people's lives that nudge them
either toward optimism or pessimism. In subsequent chapters, we will
discuss specifically how optimism translates itself into good health,
and how to encourage someone to be more of an optimist.

Optimism and Child Development

Seeking the origins of optimism and pessimism in childhood obviously
requires delving into developmental psychology, and particularly into
that field of specialty known as cognitive development. Cognitive development refers to changes in perception, intelligence, memory,
problem solving, and language across a person's lifespan. The funda-
mental premise is that children do not think as adults do: their ways of
thinking change in an orderly fashion as they become older.

Piaget's theory   The most influential theorist in cognitive development has been Jean Piaget (1896–1980). Originally trained as a biol-
ogist, with a strong interest in philosophy, Piaget[1] turned to the study
of how children think about the world. He felt that the very principles
underlying the ways in which people think develop over time. Both
the content and process of thought change.

An important Piagetian concept is the operation, defined as one
or more of the mental processes that we use to transform and manip-
ulate information. For instance, addition and subtraction are operations that make arithmetic possible. According to Piaget, the key
changes in a child's cognitive development involve the operations she
has available to her. Overall, these become more complex, more
adaptive, and more independent of immediate stimuli as she gets
older. Said another way, a child's cognitive development moves toward increasing abstraction, progressing from the concrete to the
symbolic. Earlier operations provide the foundation on which later
operations are built.

These changes take place through a child's interaction with the
world, although they also reflect her biological maturation. Piaget dis-
tinguished two general reactions to new information. Assimilation
involves modifying information to fit what is already known; accommodation, modifying what is already known to fit the information.

Suppose a young child goes to a zoo and sees a camel for the first
time. She might call it a horse, assimilating the camel to her existing
idea of a horse. Or she might call the camel a lumpy horse, and accommodate her idea of a horse to the creature standing in front of her. She
recognizes that horses seem to come in two varieties—regular and
lumpy. There is no fixed order implied here, because these operations
continually alternate in the course of a child's cognitive development.

Consider optimism and pessimism as beliefs that develop
through the assimilation and accommodation of new information,
just as all beliefs do. In some cases, new information is simply fit into
someone's habitual view of things. In other cases, it mediates changes
from an optimistic view to a pessimistic one, or vice versa.

Piaget believed that a child's available cognitive operations develop through four discrete stages. The exact times at which different
children enter or leave a given stage differ, but the sequence is regarded as invariant. With regard to each stage, we have something to
say about how optimism and pessimism develop. Consistent with
Piaget's basic premise, these ways of thinking take on different significance granted the stage.

The *sensorimotor stage* corresponds to the period from birth to about two years of age. The advances in a child's motor development allow her to explore her environment. She hits, shakes, touches, and tastes just about all of the objects she comes across. She performs many of these activities over and over again, like repeatedly dropping a spoon from her highchair. Piaget calls these repetitive behaviors circular reactions. They exemplify the general process of accommodation because the child thereby learns which of her actions are under her control and which are not (as when her mother takes the spoon away).

Circular reactions are directly pertinent to optimism as we construe it. A child's sense of efficacy (Chapter 3) may well precede her ability to think in abstract terms. Children at only two months of age react differently to events they can control and those they cannot.

For instance, Watson conducted an experiment in which he hung mobiles over the cribs of infants.[2] In one condition of this study, the mobile was connected to the infant's pillow in the crib in such a way that any time the infant moved his head, the mobile moved as well. In the other condition, the mobile moved but not in response to anything that the child did. Infants smiled and cooed more in the first condition than in the second, showing positive reactions to events over which they have control. This makes sense: even adults relish the experience of having an impact on the world.

Also during the sensorimotor stage, object permanence develops: the knowledge that objects exist even when out of sight. A simple example: an infant is propped up so that he can see an interesting object in the researcher's hand. The researcher moves her hand, and the child's eyes follow along. What happens if the researcher's hand moves behind a screen, so that the infant can no longer see the object?

In the first few months of life, once the hand and the object it holds are gone from sight, the child will not look for their reappearance. He acts as if they do not exist any more. An older infant continues to turn his head, expecting them to appear on the other side of the screen. Piaget argues from findings like this that the child must develop the idea that things continue to exist even when they cannot be seen.

Again the relevance to optimism and pessimism is clear. Notions of the future—positive or negative—cannot really be entertained until a child establishes object permanence. Prior to that the child lives in a perpetual present. We can speak of the child in this stage of cognitive development as neither optimistic nor pessimistic.

The *preoperational stage* is the second discrete period of cognitive development that Piaget identified. It occurs sometime between the ages of two and six. The paramount cognitive achievement here is that the child first starts to think symbolically. Consider these behaviors, which first appear at this time:

- children "making believe" that one object is another
- children pretending to be mother or father
- children starting to draw, intentionally representing objects on paper (or the wall, as sometimes happens)
- children reporting that they dream
- children beginning to count and understand the notion of "number"
- children using language

With the ability to represent the world in symbolic terms, the child has at his disposal a host of new cognitive skills, and finally we see optimism and pessimism akin to that of adults start to appear.

At the same time, however, he will still *not* think exactly like an adult. Children are notably egocentric, which means they can only see things from their own point of view, perceptually and otherwise. If a child is asked what his mother or father might like for a present, he will probably suggest something that he himself would like, such as a toy or a cookie. The child is not being selfish; he simply cannot grasp a perspective that is not his own.

In this stage, we start to see children showing their optimism and pessimism by making statements about the future likelihood of events. However, we should expect these statements to be unrealistically egocentric. Further, we should also expect that they may not mean the same thing to an adult that they would to a child.[3]

To amplify: research with children this age suggests that they confuse luck and skill as explanations of outcomes, using them interchangeably. They fail to appreciate the role that effort plays in achievement. And they may not distinguish between the mere association of two events and a true cause-effect relationship.

Next is the *concrete operations stage,* beginning at about age seven and lasting until about age eleven. The child's thinking during this stage becomes more logical and integrated. She can now think of objects along more than one dimension at a time. And she learns that objects can be transformed or manipulated in one way without being changed in other ways. Piaget studied a variety of examples of what is called conservation: the recognition that characteristics of objects or substances like number, length, mass, area, and volume stay the same even if their appearance changes.

For example, suppose a researcher shows a child a tall thin glass filled with milk. The same milk is then poured into a short wide glass. The researcher asks her which glass holds more milk? The tall one, says the child in the preoperational stage, because the level of milk is higher. In contrast, the child in the concrete operations stage recognizes that the milk poured into different glasses is the same. Logic and problem solving, complex skills to be sure, are finally within the child's grasp.

We believe that adult-like optimism and pessimism appear during this stage. Because the child can now see how certain actions lead to certain outcomes and not others, and because she can work backwards from outcomes to understand the actions that precede them, we expect her to hold a sophisticated view of the future and its relationship to her action or inaction in the present.

The final stage of cognitive development begins about age 12, and is called the *formal operations stage* because the child's mental processes can now regularly operate in the abstract. She can pose and answer hypothetical questions. "Large" issues like the self, love, art, friendship, justice, and the meaning of life occupy much of the adolescent's time because she is able to think about them for the first time. The world is seen not just as it is, but as it might be . . . or should be . . . or cannot be.

Optimism and pessimism are particularly relevant to the adolescent because they provide vantage points from which to examine these larger issues. It is only when we become adolescents that we develop "points of view" about which we can think. Children of course have a perspective, and this perspective is subject to many influences. But only in adolescence is the person aware of perspectives, realizing that how she sees things is possibly different than the way parents or teachers or friends see things.

We suspect that adolescence is when optimism or pessimism becomes solidified as a cognitive habit, depending on the degree to which each is entwined with the child's developing identity. During adolescence, the teenager turns away from her family as a reference and guide in favor of her peer group. Remember that we have argued all along that optimism and pessimism reflect one's surroundings. The adolescent's choice of peer groups, whether they are composed of optimistic or pessimistic individuals, critically influences her own sense of optimism or pessimism.

Conclusions We see the seeds of optimism and pessimism present in the child's first tentative exploration of the world and his ability to make it respond. It is through the circular reactions described by Piaget that the child first acquires the sense of himself as an agent. If this process is thwarted, the seeds of pessimism have been sown, because his subsequent development is rooted in a shaky sense of self.

What can further shape this sense of agency? Obviously abuse and neglect cause profound disruptions; so too may any and all sorts of losses and disappointments—especially when the child cannot understand them. Many theories of the origins of depression stress the occurrence of an early loss, particularly the loss of a parent to divorce or death. In fact, the empirical evidence in support of these theories is good.[4] At the same time, the timing of these losses is important. As a child gets older, he can start to understand what the loss means, that it is not a reflection on himself, but this can happen only after egocentrism has loosened its grip on his view of things.[5]

These are obvious points. Abuse and neglect, divorce and death—no one believes that these are healthy for children. But there is a more subtle yet no doubt more pervasive way to thwart the development of a child's optimism: inconsistency on the part of parents and teachers. Optimism and pessimism are theories about the future. They are grounded in the individual's present reality, and if the present is characterized by capriciousness, confusion, and/or chaos, then pessimism is probably a more viable theory than optimism.

Consider what inconsistency does to a child's beliefs about the future. It teaches him a series of pessimistic lessons:

- Good things today may well be gone tomorrow.
- Don't believe what other people say.
- Distrust experience.
- Actions have nothing to do with outcomes.
- Why bother with hopes and plans, schemes and dreams?

We wish that we could agree with the romantic notion that we need only step aside and let the child's "natural" optimism surface. But we think that optimism must and should be cultivated. We point out two general strategies, both necessary. The first is to provide a consistent world for the child. Then he can come to trust his environment and thereby himself. The second is to ensure positive outcomes that are due to his own efforts. We do not mean indulgences or presents or surprises but rather outcomes that the child actively earns through doing things.

Once children start to propose different sorts of explanations for bad events, then we can examine their characteristic styles of doing so. Why do some children offer optimistic explanations, whereas other children offer pessimistic ones? Following from our discussion of the sources of self-efficacy in Chapter 3, we imagine there are at least four important influences on the development of a child's explanatory style.

First are the child's actual triumphs. Success breeds success, and optimism follows in its wake. This is what we meant in Chapter 1 when we argued that optimism is reality based. It is not that adults or children cannot be optimistic when the going gets rough, but it is easier for them when the facts warrant optimism than when they do not.

Second is the nature of adult feedback. Consider the research conducted by developmental psychologist Carol Dweck. Dweck has studied how teachers respond to grade school students.[6] Suppose a child does something wrong in class. Often the teacher's criticism contains a causal explanation, which is sometimes explicit and sometimes implied:

• Oh, when will you learn to pay attention?
• You're so rowdy!
• You're never going to get this right.

Dweck's research method is to sit unobtrusively in a classroom and see how teachers evaluate what children do. She indeed finds that teachers respond differently to different students, and these children internalize this feedback and become more or less optimistic as a result. Criticism that implies a cause under the child's control—like his or her effort—ends up boosting optimism. But criticism that implies a cause about which the child can do nothing—like his or her intelligence—can undercut it.

Third is the optimism or pessimism directly displayed by those significant in the child's life. Beliefs are not always learned one piece at a time but are often assimilated as a whole. In Chapter 3, we mentioned Bandura's studies of modeling, a pervasive form of learning in which a child learns to behave in the ways that another person—the model—does.[7] Modeling provides a persuasive explanation of how we acquire many complex behavior patterns, such as aspects of attitudes and sex roles.

Modeling seems a plausible account of how we develop optimism or pessimism. If the child hears her parents being hopeful about the future, then she will be too. If the parents are gloomy, she will adopt their perspective. Children follow the example of models to the degree that they find them attractive, credible, and/or powerful—thus the possible danger of a peer group whose leader is pessimistic but charismatic.

Fourth is the extent and nature of any early trauma or disappointment. As already noted, there is a relationship between loss of one's parent to death at a young age and later susceptibility to depression. By extrapolation, perhaps early losses predispose a person to pessimism. These effects are apt to be subtle, because they depend on not just the loss per se and the age of the child, but his particular stage of cognitive development. If he is at a stage where the finality of loss can be understood, but not the fact that he himself was in no way responsible, then the grounds for pessimism may well be laid. Each subsequent loss may reinstantiate this pessimistic view, putting the child at further risk for the negative consequences of pessimism—including poor health.

Specific Investigations

We have asserted from a theoretical perspective that optimism and pessimism in the adult sense are first evident around the age of eight, when the child's cognitive development has advanced to the point where he can understand and express these sorts of expectations, and that specific experiences are associated with variations in viewpoint. (We do not mean that there are no influences on optimism or pessimism prior to the age of eight. Very early experiences are probably quite critical; it is just that their effects—on optimism and pessimism—may not be evident until years later.[8])

Studies of the appearance of optimism.   What is the empirical evidence? Researchers have discovered that age eight is when children first begin to show a range of responses to failure.[9] Earlier, most children behave in much the same way. On the face of it, their reactions would appear to be optimistic and certainly not pessimistic. But it would be more accurate to describe them as neither, because the child is not thinking ahead to a future, good or bad. Perhaps this is where the connotation of optimism with childishness comes from; but the analogy is misleading because children and adults think in very different ways.

Studies show that even in the wake of failure, most young children express extremely high expectancies when asked to predict their future performance at some task.[10] In other words, they do not realistically appraise their successes and failures.[11] And they do not experience negative feelings if they happen to fail.[12] When five- and six-year-old children are asked to say how they are doing in school, most report that they are at the very top of the class.[13]

Eight-year-olds see personality characteristics and abilities as stable and consistent. As we have seen, judgments about stability and consistency are characteristics of explanatory style and thus make optimistic or pessimistic thinking possible. Younger children do not expect people to act in consistent ways, either across different situations or across time.

A study by Susan Nolen-Hoeksema supports these generalizations. She interviewed 94 children whose ages ranged between four and eight.[14] Each child was asked to explain hypothetical events, like "a friend says he doesn't want to play with you anymore." Their explanations were scored for pessimistic versus optimistic explanatory style with the CAVE technique, described in Chapter 1. The very young children did not explain *any* of these events with causes that were internal, stable, or global. Bad events were always explained in terms of the intervention of external agents: friends, parents, and teachers. Because there was no variation in what the children said, there is no way to characterize them as more versus less optimistic.

With increasing age, children were more likely to recognize that causes could be internal—that how they behaved had something to do with what happened to them. And they were more likely to offer causes that presupposed some generality across time and outcome. In other words, their explanations invoked stable and global causes. However, not all children showed these trends, which means that there was a range of responses—the emergence of explanatory style as our earlier analysis implied.

Nolen-Hoeksema also asked the teachers of these children to rate each child on the extent to which he or she behaved in passive and helpless ways. For the older children, high scores on teacher ratings were associated with pessimism and—of course—low scores with optimism. No relationship at all was found for the younger children, suggesting that "optimistic" or "pessimistic" statements did not function the same way for them as they did for the older children.

A handful of studies have looked specifically at the sorts of early experiences and events that precede later optimism and pessimism. These studies investigated the factors we discussed earlier as possible influences on the development of optimism or pessimism: successes and triumphs versus losses and disappointments, consistency versus inconsistency, adult feedback, and modeling. After describing these studies and their results, we will draw together the common threads.

A retrospective study   With Beth Klavens and Michelle Dean, we planned and carried through an exploration of some of the early influences on optimism.[15] We limited our investigation mainly to those influences within the family and peer group.

Two limitations of this study must be acknowledged. First, we did not assess explanatory style but rather its near relative, dispositional optimism (discussed in Chapter 3). We did this because the available measure of dispositional optimism is quite brief, and we wanted to ask our research subjects as many other questions as possible in the limited amount of time we had with them. Second, the study was retrospective: we asked our subjects to recall events from their childhood. We treated what they said as valid, but we concede that the data can be second-guessed. Anyone's memory in the best of circumstances is suspect. There are matters that people cannot or will not report upon with much accuracy. This problem becomes acute when one is trying to relate differences in what people report about their childhoods to a current belief pattern (like optimism or pessimism) that arguably influences the very memories people report.

It seems reasonable to expect that optimists will report happier memories and more recollections of efficacy than pessimists—this after all is the essence of what it means to be an optimist. Optimists may well frame their childhoods more positively, after the fact, than do pessimists. Further, we know that mood influences a person's memory.[16] Someone in a good mood better remembers positive occurrences than negative ones, whereas someone in a bad mood better remembers negative occurrences than positive ones.

These difficulties are not insurmountable. What they mean is that we must take into greater account "objective" memories—such as whether one's parents were divorced—that no doubt have greater validity when recalled than more "subjective" memories in which the past is abstractly evaluated or characterized—such as whether one's parents were even-handed in discipline. Also, we should be impressed if we find that certain childhood experiences are apparently *not* related to adult optimism and pessimism, because these mean that subjects have *not* across the board rewritten history to be consistent with their current psychological states. Usually researchers are greedy. They want each of the variables measured to relate to all of the others. Here is an exception. An absence of differences in one place implies that we can have some confidence in the differences that show up elsewhere.

Our research subjects were University of Michigan students, 52 men and 73 women. We asked them to complete a questionnaire which assigned them scores reflecting their relative optimism or pessimism. Then they completed a long questionnaire ranging over events and experiences in their past.

(a) We asked about such general characteristics as their sex, age, year in school, and race. Of these, only race proved to be related to optimism. Minorities were more pessimistic than majorities. This finding makes sense given the current plight of minorities in our society.[17] Just when and how this pessimism develops we do not know, but it certainly has a basis in fact.

(b) We asked each subject, "While you were growing up, how did your mother and father usually act?" We provided six scales to rate the following traits:

• happy versus sad
• religious versus not religious
• socially withdrawn versus active
• optimistic versus pessimistic
• negative versus positive self-image
• encouraging or discouraging about hoping for the best in the future

We were trying to assess different dimensions of the subjects' memories of their parents as optimistic or pessimistic.

Most of these ratings showed a relationship to the subjects' current levels of optimism or pessimism. Optimistic individuals remembered both their mothers and their fathers as usually being happy, socially active, optimistic, having a positive self-image, and encouraging them to hope for the best. Again, these results are not surprising. A simply way to describe their thrust is to say that optimistic parents produce optimistic children; pessimistic parents produce pessimistic children. Whether or not parents were religious had no particular effect on the optimism of their children,[18] probably because religion takes so many different forms.

(c) We asked the subjects a dozen questions about how their fathers usually treated them while they were growing up. Was he comforting, encouraging, critical, or whatever? *None* of these answers was systematically related to the subject's optimism or pessimism.

When the identical questions were asked with respect to their mothers, some of their answers *were* related to the optimism versus pessimism of the subject as a young adult. Specifically, here is how the children who grew up to be optimists described their mothers' behavior:

• Mother approved when I effectively criticized someone's ideas.
• Mother did *not* say that teachers expected too little.
• Mother did *not* want to know where I was and what I was doing.
• Mother did *not* say I was a big problem.

As we see it, what is common to these answers is that mothers encouraged independence on the part of their growing children, conveyed trust, and did not undercut their education and ability to explore the world.

That fathers' treatment of subjects bore no relationship to their optimism or pessimism may simply reflect typical patterns of child-rearing in this country when the subjects were young. Mothers were more likely to be involved in the day-to-day socialization of their children. Fathers' interaction with their children may have been too infrequent to have as much impact as mothers'.

(d) As we have been saying, optimism resides in a social context. It thus seemed plausible that one of the origins of optimism might lie in satisfying relationships with other people, so we asked subjects about the sorts of friendships they had when they were growing up. The sheer number of close friends they once had was not related to optimism or pessimism, but the number of these early friends who were still close to the subject did prove important. Optimists had more friends remaining from childhood than did pessimists, implying that continuity of friendship is more important than the absolute number at any given moment.

Interestingly, pessimists were somewhat more likely than optimists to have had a best friend while growing up. At first glance, one would think that having a best friend would be a healthy experience, cultivating optimism. This result is therefore contrary to the obvious prediction. But perhaps its significance becomes clear in light of the other data. Pessimists did not experience continuity in friendship, which means that when they—so to speak—put all their eggs in the one basket represented by a best friend, they fell out along the way to adulthood. It may not be an exaggeration to say that when young people lose touch with a best friend, they feel betrayed, and pessimism may follow.

This interpretation is consistent with our remaining findings about childhood friendship. Optimists were more likely than pessimists to report that they were "totally" satisfied with the companionship and emotional reassurance their friends provided them. We also asked about two other possible functions of social support—information and practical help—but these showed no relationship to optimism or pessimism. This suggests that the sort of friendship that encourages optimism is not a utilitarian, practical relationship but rather an emotional one.

(e) We asked subjects about their brothers or sisters. There was no relationship between optimism and pessimism and the size of one's family. Neither was there any relationship between optimism and pessimism and one's birth order in the family—oldest, middle, or youngest.

Among those subjects who had at least one brother or sister (and these constituted the vast majority of our sample), some interesting results emerged in relation to what we can call sibling rivalry. Optimists reported that they were seldom compared to their brothers or sisters; pessimists in contrast reported that they were constantly compared. Further, optimists rarely wanted to trade places with a brother or sister, whereas pessimists much more frequently remembered this as a wish. Similarly, optimists were not as apt to be jealous of their brothers or sisters as were pessimists. Taken together, these results suggest that optimism originates in a family in which comparisons among children are not made, and each child feels satisfied to be who she or he is. Resentment and envy foreshadow pessimism, which makes perfect sense.

A fascinating finding emerged from these questions about sibling rivalry and resentment. We further asked with whom the subject wanted to trade places—if that were ever a wish—and of whom the subject felt jealous—again, if that emotion had been experienced. Pessimists wanted to trade places with a younger brother or sister; they were jealous of them. Optimists said just the opposite. To the degree that they wanted to trade places with a sibling, it was with an older one. To the degree that they were jealous of a sibling, it was an older brother or sister who was their rival.

It is interesting to try to sort out these patterns from the viewpoint of a child. One very obvious fact of life to a child is that the social world is age-graded:

• Wait until you are older.
• That's just for big kids.
• You can do that next year.

Most of us remember our parents saying these kinds of things.

What does it mean to be jealous of an older brother or sister? It means that one can aspire to be like the older sibling when one is older. A child may be impatient, but he or she knows the time will come.

And what does it mean to be jealous of a younger brother or sister? In this case the passage of time is irrelevant, because one can never be younger. Even children know this, and the younger brother or sister of whom they are resentful will always be younger, no matter how long they wait. That is depressing, we would think, and the translation of this gloomy state of affairs into pessimism in young adulthood seems inevitable.

(f) In Chapter 6, we will document a strong relationship in adults between optimism and active coping in the face of bad events. Does this relationship have a developmental trajectory? Accordingly, we asked our subjects to think back to when they were growing up and bad things happened to them. How did they usually respond? We queried them about a number of possible coping strategies. Only one of these showed no relationship to later optimism or pessimism, probably because it is something children often have trouble doing: putting things out of their mind. Indeed, this was the least frequently chosen alternative.

However, every other coping strategy showed a sensible relationship with our measure of dispositional optimism. Specifically, we found that optimists, when compared to pessimists, were as children *more likely:*

• to understand their feelings
• to seek out more information

- to try to find solutions
- to look on the bright side of things
- to turn to other people
- to understand why bad things happened

At the same time optimists, when compared to pessimists, were as children *less likely:*

- to become angry
- to become depressed

As the twig is bent, so grows the tree. Children's patterns of coping may lead to characteristic worldviews, optimistic or pessimistic, which in turn may influence the patterns of coping they show as adults.

(g) We also asked our subjects about the goals they had set for themselves in the past that they had expected to achieve by the present time. We requested that they think of up to five such goals. For each, our subjects indicated whether or not they had achieved the goal and how difficult it had been for them to do so. There was a very slight link between achieving goals and being optimistic, but this was nowhere as robust a relationship as the one between finding one's goals easy to achieve and being optimistic. In other words, pessimists found it difficult to achieve their goals, although they eventually did reach them.

Let us not overinterpret these findings, because we do not know if the optimists and pessimists in our sample pursued the same or different goals. But to the extent that we can take the patterns at face value, they challenge the way we think about the values of striving in the face of difficulty. We usually profess to respect the person who has to work harder than others for the same achievement. But our findings suggest that for the individual who finds the pursuit of goals strenuous, the difficulty can take a toll on his or her optimism.

All university instructors know that some students work long and diligently in order to get a B in a course. Other students breeze through without attending class and without doing much reading. They take an exam and earn the same grade of B. Although we have not made a systematic study, we would bet the former students eventually get discouraged.[19] Yes, the goal of a decent grade has been met, but look at the cost! "It doesn't seem fair!" these students invariably say. We concur, but it is often the way the world works. Effort is not rewarded to the degree that achievement is.

(h) Finally, we asked the subjects about stressful events in the past year. Here we were interested in more recent influences on optimism. We presented them with a variety of events that might affect their characteristic optimism or pessimism and asked them which (if any) had actually occurred. Not all of the events showed a systematic relationship to their optimism or pessimism. However, there were a handful of events that did. Optimists, when compared to pessimists, were:

- less likely to have held a job while attending college
- less likely to have committed a minor violation of the law
- less likely to have changed to a different line of work
- less likely to have had a change in their responsibilities at work
- more likely to have had an outstanding personal achievement
- more likely to have taken a trip or vacation

These particular findings are inherently ambiguous, precisely because they occurred in the relatively recent past. We cannot know whether these events influenced the subjects' optimism or pessimism, or the reverse, or both. These results may reflect the operation of a third factor, like socioeconomic status, which influences both optimism and life events. Because the subjects in this study were college students, the events about which we asked may have different significance than analogous occurrences in the lives of working adults. Still, we can conclude that optimism goes hand in hand with achievement and good feelings, while pessimism is associated with trouble and hassle.

A prospective study   We now turn to a second investigation of childhood influences on adult optimism and pessimism. With Joel Weinberger and David McClelland of Boston University, we undertook a prospective study of how different approaches to child-rearing are associated with optimism or pessimism in adults. This study is much more solid than our retrospective study, because we did not have to rely on the memory of research subjects to reconstruct their pasts.

The study itself began in the late 1940s. Robert Sears, Eleanor Maccoby, and Harry Levin, the original investigators, extensively interviewed several hundred mothers, mostly from the northeast of the

United States, about how they raised their children, then five years old.[20]

About four decades passed, and then we picked up the study. The original children were now middle-aged adults. Ninety of them were recontacted, and they consented to complete measures for us. Among the things they did was to write a brief essay describing the worst events that had recently befallen them. We used the CAVE procedure to ascertain their characteristic optimism or pessimism.[21]

From the earlier efforts of Sears, Maccoby, and Levin, we knew how these adults were treated as children. It was therefore possible for us to ask what childhood experiences preceded optimism and to have confidence in the validity of the results we thereby obtained.

Table 4–1 shows the major factors that foreshadowed optimism. The list of predisposing factors is long, but the picture proves quite consistent and coherent. Children from happy homes—where harshness was absent—were more likely to be optimistic. Avoiding disappointments also proved important for optimism to blossom later. The single strongest predictor of adult pessimism was a child's failure to succeed at early bowel training, before the age of twelve months. The role of the mother was more important than that of the father, again reflecting the social realities of time and place.

We need to make some qualifications here. First, many factors were examined; not all of them bore a significant relationship to adult optimism versus pessimism. Second, this research was conducted in a different era, so as in any developmental study, there may be some historically specific considerations that should make us cautious about generalizing the findings. Third, the original researchers had primarily psychoanalytic concerns; hence their interest in questions about toilet training, weaning, and discipline. That a number of these aspects of child-rearing bear relationships to adult optimism and pessimism is interesting, but may reflect other characteristics of socialization with which these were correlated.[22]

The findings of this study are nonetheless quite consistent—at the appropriate level of abstraction—with the results from the retrospective study. This is scientifically encouraging, because the studies were different in detail, and the subjects were from different generations. Indeed, our college student subjects could well have been the children of the subjects in the Sears et al. investigation.

Two studies of parents and their children   We want to describe a few more bits of evidence concerning the origins of optimism. If the mod-

TABLE 4–1. *Childhood Influences on Adult Optimism*

Optimism was more likely among adults when 40 years previously:

- their mothers had high-status jobs, as opposed to low-status jobs (or no job at all)
- they did not watch a lot of television
- they were not separated from their mothers during the first nine months of life (separations at later times showed no relationship)
- they were not cared for by anyone but their mothers during infancy
- they did not cry a lot
- they took a short time to be weaned
- their mothers did not use punishment (like spanking) during weaning
- their mothers made no early unsuccessful attempts at bowel training
- they showed a mild response to toilet training
- their mothers placed few restrictions on how they could play in the house
- their mothers used little pressure to make them conform to restrictions
- their mothers placed few restrictions on their physical mobility
- their mothers did not expect instant obedience from them
- they were not clingy
- they were independent
- their mothers encouraged them to be sociable
- their mothers did not permit inappropriate aggression toward other children
- their mothers did not severely punish them for aggression against their parents
- they did not act aggressively toward their parents
- they were not spanked frequently
- they were not ridiculed by their mother as a way of discipline
- they were punished consistently—parents followed through on threats to discipline
- they were not disciplined by their father in ways that their mother objected to

eling hypothesis is viable, we would expect that children should resemble significant others in their lives with respect to optimism or pessimism. A study we have conducted indeed supports this hypothesis.[23]

We administered to 96 grade school children a child's measure of explanatory style (the Children's Attributional Style Questionnaire). We also asked their parents to complete the ASQ. The results were straightforward. Optimistic mothers had optimistic children; pessimistic mothers had pessimistic children. The explanatory style of fathers and their children did not line up in this way, and so we have another example of how mothers are more directly important in socializing optimism or pessimism than are fathers. Again, the likely reason is that in typical American families, mothers spend more time with children than do fathers.[24]

This particular correlation between the optimism and pessimism of mothers and their children has been replicated by Nolen-Hoeksema in children as young as eight years old.[25] Thus, the direction of influence would indeed seem to run mostly from mother to child, rather than vice versa, because an eight-year-old has just developed adultlike optimism or pessimism. Of course there will be a mutual influence between the mother and the child with respect to optimism and pessimism, particularly as the child becomes older. But the fact that the convergence between them occurs just as the child begins to show a characteristic worldview suggests that the mothers' influence is primary.

A study by Anne Vanden Belt further shows how parental optimism or pessimism can affect the child.[26] She was interested in exploring the contribution of parental beliefs to the failure of some students to work up to their potential in the classroom. In particular, she wondered if the explanatory style of parents related to their children's academic performance and adjustment.

Approximately 100 grade school children, ages six to twelve, and their parents participated in the study. Parents—usually mothers—completed a measure of explanatory style asking them how they would explain various bad events that might befall their child. The teachers of these children then rated their classroom performance, relative to their apparent potential, along a variety of dimensions. The results were straightforward and striking. Those parents who explained bad events involving their children with internal, stable, and global causes had children who consistently failed to live up to their potential.

An immediate objection to the conclusion we wish to draw from this study, that parental explanatory style influences a child's class-room performance, is that the direction of causality actually might run in the opposite direction, from classroom performance to parental explanations. But we do not think this is a good argument.

By design, Vanden Belt included in her sample a number of students with physical and mental handicaps. If "reality" in the form of actual student performance dictated the way parents explained events involving their children, surely the parents of handicapped students would view matters more negatively than parents of nondisabled students. However, the pattern of results was exactly the same in both groups; for both disabled and nondisabled students, parental explanatory style predicted a child's classroom performance to the same degree. Presumably these beliefs are transmitted to the children, who live up (or down) to them.

A study of educational challenge   The final study we want to discuss was an investigation of how an enriched environment influences the development of a sense of optimism.[27] Specifically, we tracked the effects of an intervention in a school system that tried to boost the optimism of students.

The most direct way to combat pessimism is to eradicate the situational factors that produce it and create a setting conducive to optimism. There *must* be adequate rewards available in a setting. We are not speaking exclusively of a school's physical plant and material goods. High-tech innovations are neither necessary nor sufficient for an enriched school environment. Indeed, the most important part of the environment is other people. Students and teachers must be responsive to each other. And rewards must be contingent on what a student does, as we emphasized earlier in the chapter. There needs to be a clear connection between what one does and what ensues.

Accordingly, we worked in conjunction with a program in a junior high school that attempted to bolster the sense of efficacy among students in the "middle" of the class ranks. These children performed neither exceptionally well nor exceptionally badly. Mainly they were passive, merely going through the motions at school, creating no waves and reaching no heights.

The school system devised a program for these students that enriched their school environment in just the way we have sketched. The major innovation was to have the different classroom teachers of the students meet together daily, coordinating their lesson plans as well as team-teaching various classes. The goal was to make the different parts of the curriculum cohere and to provide a series of integrated challenges for each individual student. If one student showed a flair for numbers in math class, for example, then this information would be passed on to the social studies teacher, who would ask the student to prepare a report stressing statistics.

Our role in the project was to evaluate whether its goal of boosting the students' sense of optimism was met. We administered to the students measures of explanatory style before and after the year-long program, as well as to a comparison group of students. We found that the program was a success in encouraging students to explain events more optimistically. Whether this change led to long-term benefits—particularly with regard to the physical health of these students—is still under investigation. Sadly, the comparison group—students not in this special program—showed an erosion in their optimism over the course of the school year.

A Recipe for Producing Optimistic Children

Given the results of studies investigating the origins of optimism, we feel confident about one conclusion: optimism is a social product. If we want to see the next generation more optimistic than this one, we need to work at creating a social environment in which optimism will thrive. Here is a recipe, therefore, that parents or teachers can follow if they wish to inculcate optimism:

1. Be consistent.
2. Be positive.
3. Be responsive.
4. "Program" the children's world to be consistent, positive, and responsive.
5. Give them responsibility and encourage their independence.
6. Set realistic goals.
7. Involve them in many activities.
8. Make sure these activities are age-appropriate.
9. Get them to discriminate failures from one another.
10. Get them to generalize successes.
11. Encourage problem solving.
12. Recast failure as a challenge.
13. Encourage humor as a coping strategy.
14. Model realistic optimism for them.

15. Challenge their pessimistic views.
16. Screen their peers and teachers as best you can.

Optimism and the Child's Conception of Health

This chapter has thus far focused on the origins of optimism. In subsequent chapters, we detail exactly how the sense of optimism or pessimism engendered by childhood experiences ends up influencing adult health. But first we will take a brief look at children's notions of health. It is important to remember Piaget's premise that children think very differently than adults do. We need to encourage health among children quite differently than we do among adults.

Developmental psychologists have undertaken numerous studies to see exactly how children think about physical health and illness. Children's conceptions reflect the stage of cognitive development in which they happen to find themselves. Here are some generalizations from this literature.[28]

Young children do not perceive any association between health and illness. Further, each is described in general, nonspecific terms. Health is regarded as an enabling condition that subsumes a host of positive states and desires. When asked questions like "What does the word health mean?" or "What does it feel like to be healthy?" children younger than the age of eight give answers like:

- I can do what I want to.
- I feel happy.
- I know I am healthy because I'm in school.

Illness in contrast is thought of as a rough grouping of bad events and feelings. Some children equate being ill with being morally bad.

Children do not discern a link between internal cues and sensations and the concepts of health and illness. Presumably, they must learn what it means to feel ill and feel healthy. Of course, children are healthy or ill, but their *understanding* of what these notions entail must develop, through processes of assimilation and accommodation, just as any form of understanding must develop. Younger children have no idea about how the body works, and thus can give no particularly good rationale for how illness comes about or how it might be combated. In particular, younger children do not see a relationship between their behavior and their physical health.

Among children, a sense of vulnerability to illness is *negatively* related to preventive health behavior—like eating well or brushing one's teeth. In other words, children who are ill or believe themselves at risk for illness are less likely to behave in healthful ways. This is an interesting finding. In Chapter 6, we will discuss the safer-sex practices of gay men at risk for AIDS. Among the pessimistic, the greater a man's perceived risk for AIDS, the fewer precautions he takes. In adults, we have no trouble branding this fatalistic. In children, it reflects a lack of understanding of what cause-effect relationships are all about. However, this is not a trivial set of mistaken beliefs, because they may sow the seeds for later fatalism in the realm of health promotion.

Even when children grasp the general idea of health, they may misunderstand the particulars. Wilkinson points out that some children appreciate the idea of contagion in that illness is something that they catch from being in contact with others.[29] But at least some children assimilate the notion of contagion to the concept of the common childhood game of "It!" In other words, the person with a disease is "It!" and can give the disease to another person by tagging him or her, literally or metaphorically. So far this is a sensible view. But they may further think that once the tag has been made, the original person with the disease is no longer "It!" because the disease has been passed on.[30]

Our formula linking optimism to good health through such intermediaries as active health promotion and coping in the face of illness simply does not apply to children. More bluntly, as the developmental researcher Janet Natapoff puts it, "Teaching young children principles of health maintenance to prevent illness is meaningless."[31] We hasten to say that children should be taught healthful practices, but we cannot give them a "health" rationale in so doing and expect it to be effective. Instead, we should model healthful behaviors for them, setting examples that they can readily follow.

Some health-conscious parents we know are proceeding in ignorance of this principle. Consider the following exchange, which took place at a picnic attended by many people, some of whom brought along rich desserts:

PARENT: What is that?
CHILD: Cake!
PARENT: And what do we say about cake?
CHILD: Tastes yucky!
PARENT: What else?
CHILD: Makes you sick!

The problem here is that the child has never tasted cake in his entire life. What happens when he eventually tries it and perhaps finds it quite tasty? He will not be capable of understanding why something that tastes good might make him feel bad. The child will experience a credibility gap with regard to his parents' teachings, not only about cake but other matters.

Parents and teachers should do their best to encourage optimism among children in the ways we have sketched. They should also encourage healthful practices among children via modeling. But the young child's cognitive abilities are insufficient for one set of teachings to buttress the other. It is necessary to wait until the child is old enough to appreciate cause-effect relationships before offering health as a rationale for health-promoting activities.

5

From Optimism to Health: Biological and Emotional Routes

If the brain were so simple that we could understand it, we would be so simple we couldn't.

— *Emerson M. Pugh*

In Chapter 2, we described several studies using diverse methods which showed that optimistic thinking is associated with good health and pessimistic thinking with poor health. In Chapter 3, we further supported this association by reviewing a number of lines of research by other investigators showing more generally that "positive" psychological states are associated with good physical health. And in Chapter 4, we speculated about the origins of optimistic thinking, looking to events and experiences in childhood.

In this chapter, we begin to consider *how* optimism and pessimism might affect our health. We will talk in terms of routes, to convey the notion that people play an active role in getting from here (optimism) to there (good health). Many routes will be examined, which is not surprising, because there are innumerable influences for us to discern.

This chapter will be devoted to describing pathways *inside* the person: physiological and emotional processes. We will survey research that shows how optimism is related to these processes, and how these in turn give rise to good or bad health. In the next chapter, we will continue our discussion of routes by talking about those *outside* the person. This is a somewhat arbitrary way to divide matters, because "internal" and "external" factors mutually affect each other. But for simplicity's sake, we will go along with this rough distinction.

In particular, we will stress how people's mundane behaviors can promote or damage their health. We hope thereby to build a bridge between our research on optimistic thinking and the enormous literature on health promotion—diets, exercise programs, stress management, and the like.[1] Health promotion has sometimes been pushed upon the public in a mindless way, in at least two senses. First, an overall theory of well-being is often lacking. Instead, a "more is better" approach often encourages people to ruin their physical and emotional health in order to appear fit.[2] An overarching view of what it means to be healthy might restore some sense to health promotion in this regard.

Second, health promotion efforts understandably emphasize the body, but there is a curious neglect of the mind. Our psychological state is not simply a byproduct of our physical state, as health promotion experts often seem to imply. The influence runs in both directions.[3] Any news stand will abound with articles asserting that running will improve self-esteem. We think that self-esteem can improve running. Indeed, we want to put the mind into health promotion in a literal way, and to argue that the process of bolstering one's well-being must *start* with thoughts and beliefs.

Learned Helplessness

Some of the most intriguing research that bears on the physiological and emotional influences on health has used animals as research subjects, in the learned helplessness tradition. As we noted in Chapter 1, our current research program on explanatory style and physical well-being began in this tradition. It may seem unusual that we are speaking first about dogs and rats and mice and even goldfish. But investigations of creatures like these imply important things about creatures like us. Most importantly, these investigations lead us to appreciate how physiological and emotional processes can thwart our good health, making illness and even death more likely.

Let us turn back the clock to see what was going on in a psychological laboratory at the University of Pennsylvania more than two decades ago, where animal learning was being studied. A dog was held immobile in a harness. Brief bursts of electric shock, painful but not harmful, were delivered to the dog's legs through attached electrodes. The shocks came without a signal, and they arrived on a random schedule: 64 shocks over sixty minutes. The dog could do nothing to avoid or escape the shocks because of the harness. Once released, the dog bounded away.

The next day, the dog was placed in a long and narrow box with a wire floor and a low barrier in the middle. A shock was delivered through the floor of the box. If the dog jumped over the barrier, the shock would be turned off. If the dog failed to make this particular response, then the shock would stay on for a total of five seconds. The process was repeated again and again.

The typical dog placed in this box readily learns to jump the barrier and turn off the shock. It does so quickly and efficiently, so much so that this is a typical way that psychologists interested in rudimentary learning go about studying it. The "shuttle box" is a standard part of their laboratory equipment.

Imagine, then, the surprise of the experimental psychologists who placed the dog previously immobilized and given shocks into the shuttle box. This animal did nothing when the shock was turned on. Instead, it sat there and endured the shock. Other aspects of the dog's behavior were striking as well. Usually, when a dog is shocked like this, it shows overt signs of being upset—it whines and whimpers, it urinates, and it defecates. Instead, the dog simply sat passively with no overt signs of emotion. After repeated shocks were delivered, the dog would occasionally amble across the barrier, terminating the shock. For a normal dog, crossing the barrier would be a sure sign that the "escape response" has been learned, and one would expect it to be repeated on subsequent occasions when the shock is turned on. But this dog did not follow one escape response with another. Instead, the next time that the shock was turned on, it again sat there without moving.

The three psychologists involved in this research—Steve Maier, Bruce Overmier, and Martin Seligman—might have ignored this surprising behavior. After all, they had been interested in another problem altogether,[4] and the dog sitting there in the shuttle box was not very useful to their study. But they were good scientists, and they were struck by the dog's unusual behavior. What was going on? Why should an animal previously exposed to shocks it could not control later behave passively and indifferently when exposed to shocks that it could control?

A glib answer might be that the creature had somehow been traumatized and could not respond because its body had been damaged. But this was not the case here. The dog had experienced pain the previous day, but there was clearly no injury or trauma. The dog was perfectly capable of performing the escape response; indeed, it occasionally did so, although profiting not the least when it did. No, something else was going on.

These observations were made in the middle 1960s, when the study of cognition was accelerating.[5] So these psychologists gave a cognitive interpretation to the phenomenon they had just observed. Perhaps the dog had learned in the first place, while immobilized in the harness and given shocks, that nothing it did mattered. Regardless of the responses it did or did not make, the shocks came. The dog learned a particular expectation—that responses and outcomes had no relationship to each other.

It carried this expectation with it into the second situation, the shuttle box, where responses and outcomes were related. If the barrier were crossed, the shock would be turned off. However, the dog's expectation about what would happen in the future created passivity and emotional apathy. Further, this expectation even interfered with learning that a particular response did have an effect. The dog became oblivious to contrary evidence. Even though it was in a position to "test reality" in this new situation, the previous lesson in futility was strong enough to preclude the evidence.

The phenomenon orginally observed by these psychologists has come to be known as *learned helplessness,* because the animal "learns" an expectation in the first situation that produces "helplessness" in the second. The explanation of this phenomenon in terms of an expectation of response-outcome independence has come to be known as the learned helplessness model. Let us make some general points about learned helplessness, the phenomenon and the model, because—as we have already explained—our concern with optimism and health eventually evolved from this work.

Many studies support the contention that the learned helplessness phenomenon is produced by an expectation of response-outcome independence.[6] Alternative explanations in terms of trauma, blatant or subtle, have been ruled out. For instance, suppose we take a dog (or rat or mouse or even a goldfish) and immobilize it in the harness. We deliver shocks to it, but this time we arrange matters so that the animal can turn its nose and press a lever that turns off the shock after it has begun. Here we have arranged things so that the animal's responses do have an effect on outcomes (the shocks). This animal does not act in a helpless fashion when later placed in a shuttle box (or shuttle aquarium).

Indeed, in an elegant research design, we can keep track of the amount and the pattern of shock the animal in the situation just described actually experiences before it presses the lever. Then we can deliver exactly the same shocks to another animal, "yoked" to the first. The only difference between the two is that the first animal controls the offset of the shocks, and the second animal does not. But this difference proves critical in producing learned helplessness in the second animal but not in the first.

Let us clear up a possible misunderstanding. The animal in the harness does not simply learn to hold still. Rather, it learns that *nothing it does makes any difference*—whether holding still or moving. It is simply the nature of living things that this expectation translates itself into passivity. But the passivity per se is not directly learned. Steve Maier clarified this point in a clever study, in which the animals in the first situation were taught that they could turn off shocks delivered to them if they simply did not move.[7] If learned helplessness were a matter of directly learning to be passive, then these animals should have been particularly "helpless" when later placed in the shuttle box. But this was not the case; they readily learned the "active" response of jumping the barrier.

Cognitive theorizing about what dogs and rats learned was new in the 1960s, even controversial. For Maier, Overmier, and Seligman to suggest a cognitive interpretation of the dogs' behavior—and to call it helplessness, which was anthropomorphic, to say the least—was to throw down a challenge to conventional ways of thinking about what and how animals learned. As it turned out, learned helplessness proved impossible, or at least spectacularly awkward, to explain without referring to mental states, and so the cognitive language survived.

Learned helplessness in people   Helplessness in people is more complex than helplessness in animals, of course, because people can think in much more sophisticated ways. Still, the learned helplessness phenomenon has been demonstrated in laboratory studies with human beings, where more benign events than electric shocks—usually problems that cannot be solved—are substituted, but with the identical effects on later behavior. Following uncontrollability, a person is emotionally and behaviorally passive, and inattentive to evidence to the contrary.

Continued studies of helplessness in people led to the conclusion that other factors influenced the relationship between uncontrollability and helplessness, which was not as automatic as the helplessness model makes it seem. Particularly important was how a person explained the causes of an uncontrollable event. These causes seemed to set the parameters for his subsequent helplessness following uncontrollable events. Some causal explanations were more likely than others to produce pervasive helplessness. And these explanations are the ones we describe as internal, stable, and global, in other words, pessimistic ones. The opposite types of explanation, invoking external, unstable, and specific causes, are not so apt to produce helplessness, and these are thus optimistic ones.

Explanatory style, as we made clear in Chapter 1, is important because it influences the particular explanations for uncontrollable events that befall a person; these particular explanations in turn set the parameters for his or her expectations about later events; these expectations then determine the way someone behaves in the wake of the uncontrollable events, helplessly or vigorously.[8]

The link between learned helplessness and optimism should now be clear. Both entail an expectation for the future. An optimistic expectation is that events can be controlled in the future, that responses will bear a relationship to outcomes. In contrast, a pessimistic expectation is that events will elude control in the future, that responses will bear no relationship to outcomes.

The uncontrollability of the original events is critical. Uncontrollability is unambiguously a psychological notion, because it refers to a transaction between an individual and her environment that cannot be reduced to another—i.e., physiological—level. Although the exact manner in which the helpless animal or person represents the expectation of uncontrollability is not known, this representation must be psychological, and it must be central.

One of the intriguing implications of the helplessness model is that events need not be negative in order to produce helplessness. What is important, again, is simply their uncontrollability, which means that noncontingent rewards can make a person helpless. Seligman discussed several examples of depression among highly fortunate individuals:

Depressed, successful people tell you that they are now rewarded not for what they're doing, but for who they are or what they *have* done. Having achieved the goal that they strove for, their rewards now come independently of any ongoing instrumental activity. There are more depressed and suicidal beautiful women than it seems there should be; few people get more rewards: attention, cars, love. What they disgustedly say when reminded how fortunate they are is: "I got these things for what I look like, not for what I really am."[9]

We must point out that success-induced helplessness and depression prove rare, because most people have a strong tendency to see rewards as something that they have brought about through their own efforts, even when the role of chance is made clear![10] But even these few examples prove of interest, for showing how important it is for someone to have a sense of control over important events. When this sense of control is shaken, even though the person is materially well off, a psychological toll is taken.

Applications of learned helplessness   The learned helplessness model has attracted the attention of psychologists who wish to explain why people act in a passive, maladaptive way. When we see a person behaving listlessly, failing to engage the world and voicing negative expectations, we may ask if learned helplessness is at work. Has the person experienced a history of uncontrollable events? Does he expect no link between what he does and what happens to him? Is the setting in which he acts helplessly indeed one that would be responsive to his active efforts? If we can answer yes to these questions, we can conclude that learned helplessness may be responsible for his plight.[11]

We have elsewhere catalogued several dozen applications of the learned helplessness model: to academic failure, to burnout in the helping professions, to alcoholism, to "choking" in athletic contests, to battered women, to abused children, to the effects of institutionalization, and so on, and so forth.[12] One of our favorite applications started with the premise that people could become helpless in a vicarious fashion—by watching uncontrollable events happen to other people. This premise is a special case of the general learning process called modeling.[13]

So, Grace Ferrari Levine carried out a content analysis of television newscasts during the 1970s.[14] Five-minute segments on NBC and

CBS were coded according to the degree of helplessness that was evident:

4 = central figure completely unable to affect outcomes
3 = central figure mostly unable to affect outcomes
2 = central figure somewhat able to control outcomes
1 = central figure able to affect outcomes but did not do so
0 = irrelevant; or central figure completely affects outcomes

For example, catastrophes like airplane crashes or earthquakes were assigned a score of 4, whereas athletic victories due to skilled performances were scored 0.

Results showed that fully 14% of news segments were given the highest helplessness scores, followed by 19% in the second highest category. No consistent differences between the two networks were found, although Levine observed that the "same" story as covered on both networks frequently received different scores, suggesting that helplessness as modeled on television news does not reside solely in the news event itself, but in the way it is covered.

Levine's study is more of a tickler than anything else. We can only conclude from it that uncontrollable bad events impinge on television viewers every night. What is unknown is the effect of these events, and whether the 1970s were a particularly helpless era or not. We wish that newscasts of the 1960s had been compared with those from the 1970s. And now that we are through the 1980s, we wish that contemporary newscasts could be included in these comparisons as well. With problems such as environmental pollution becoming more complex, the apparent futility of individual effort may become more pronounced.

Learned helplessness researchers are drawn to investigations such as this one by a desire to understand people's problems and how to devise solutions to them. In the course of this research, a great deal has been learned about helplessness and its predisposing cognitive state, pessimism. By the logic of this research, everything learned about pessimism is also something learned about optimism, because these function as psychological opposites. If pessimism has a particular consequence, then optimism has the opposite consequence. If pessimism has a given antecedent, then optimism has the opposite antecedent. Only recently have those of us who work within the learned helplessness tradition turned our explicit attention to optimism, although we have in effect been studying it all along.

Physiological Routes

We have discussed the learned helplessness phenomenon because it leads us into an understanding of the physiological processes by which optimism and pessimism are linked to good and bad health, respectively. The researchers who originally discovered the phenomenon in dogs, and particularly Steve Maier, have taken ever closer looks at the physiological aspects of learned helplessness. The earliest research here did not focus on these because it was important to show that trauma in the original situation did not produce helplessness in the second. This would trivialize the phenomenon. (Indeed, a tongue-in-cheek article written at this time proposed that dead pigeons were particularly likely to act in a passive way following shocks.[15]) Accordingly, studies were engineered to rule out any biological explanation and show that the phenomenon was a psychological one.

In retrospect, this rigid distinction between psychology and biology is a false dichotomy, a point we will discuss further in Chapter 8. No doubt Steve Maier was correct in trying first to establish learned helplessness as a psychological phenomenon, one produced by learning expectations and not by brutal physiological trauma. Once learned helplessness was accepted as psychologically real, however, Maier reminded everyone that it is a biological phenomenon as well.[16]

In a series of studies by Steve Maier and other researchers,[17] the following discoveries were made about helpless animals (i.e., those exposed to uncontrollable shocks) and thus by extrapolation about helpless people (i.e., those with pessimistic expectations):

- These creatures are analgesic; in other words, painful stimuli like electric shocks do not hurt them as much as they hurt animals not previously exposed to uncontrollable shocks.
- This analgesic effect is brought about by increased endorphins—the naturally produced substances in the body that mimic the effect of opiates, letting us "turn off" extreme pain we may experience.
- A point of fact: too many endorphins can interfere with the effective functioning of the immune system, because they lodge in it and suppress its ability to fight off foreign invaders.[18]
- Indeed, helpless animals show immunosuppression.
- And helpless animals are more susceptible to tumor growth.

Note that we have all the plot elements for a coherent story about how optimism makes good health more likely, told in biological language.

A sense of control can forestall the sequence of harmful consequences that start with uncontrollable events. What happens if this
sequence is allowed to run on without interruption? See Figure 5–1.
Remember the critical role played here by one's expectations.

This figure diagrams as good an explanation of how minds and
bodies are connected as any that have been proposed since they were
first split into two different realms (Chapter 8). Nothing in this hypothesized sequence is implausible; each step has been shown in animals. And if it unfolds in animals, it should in people. Many of the
steps have been empirically confirmed. We know, for instance, that
uncontrollable life events take a toll on someone's immune system.[19]
We know that such events make illness more likely.[20] And so on.

Not mentioned so far is the time scale involved, and the route
sketched in Figure 5–1 has no mileage markers. Because these physiological events take place on a cellular level, and because they may do
so very quickly, we suspect that the sequence must be played out time
and again before it has a marked effect on anyone's health. One uncontrollable event will probably not result in illness for an individual.
It is the chronicity of these events that stamps in the route.

Let us offer some qualifications. In contrast to animals, our "expectations" bear no one-to-one relationship with the events we experience. This is why we choose to look at explanatory style, as a

FIGURE 5–1. An Explanation of How Minds and Bodies Are Connected

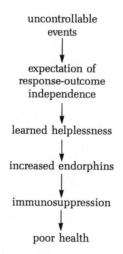

summary of someone's expectations. Some of the studies cited above prove difficult to replicate. No one that we know has declared the original studies flukes, but the point is probably that these physiological links are fragile ones, at least as they have been studied, and they may depend on subtle aspects of the experimental procedure.[21]

There are in principle many other physiological routes that lead from cognition to health. The route we have been discussing is charted through the immune system. But another route might go through the adrenal system and end up putting a strain on the heart. For example, we know that uncontrollable events are more stressful than controllable ones, so perhaps the body's emergency system is engaged too often among the helpless, eventually causing it to give out. Remember the possible relationships we sketched in Chapter 3 between pessimism and the Type A behavior pattern.

And making things even more complicated is that a person's level of stress apparently affects how her body deals with cholesterol.[22] In other words, it is not simply how much cholesterol a person consumes—it is what happens to it once it is in her system, and if her body is under stress, she will end up with a higher cholesterol level. Needless to say, the interrelationships of the different systems of the body are vastly rich, which means that what we are calling different routes really are not. Perhaps a more satisfactory metaphor here is to call these different stories.

James Dabbs, a researcher at the University of Georgia, recently told us of an intriguing correlation in a sample of male college students between explanatory style and testosterone level. The more optimistic individuals had higher levels of male sex hormone than the more pessimistic ones. What does this mean? We can only speculate, and certainly the finding needs replication. But perhaps the physiological pathway between optimism and health might be hormonal as well.[23] And perhaps this has something to do with the sex difference in health.

We conclude by saying that there is good evidence for at least one physiological pathway running from optimism to health: through the immune system. We can generate a number of testable predictions that follow from the hypothesizing of this path. To begin with, optimists and pessimists should be differentially vulnerable to infectious diseases. And they should have different levels of circulating endorphins. They should variously do the sorts of things that we know people with different levels of endorphins do.

But we do not want to put all of our explanatory eggs in a biological basket. We are not biological reductionists, and we think there is every reason to look for additional routes between optimism and health. It is of course important to remember that these different routes may constantly intersect with each other.

Emotional Routes

One of the best-established links in the entire psychological literature is the association between explanatory style and depression. Literally hundreds of investigations have reported an association between pessimistic explanations for bad events and increases in one's depressive symptoms—in children, young adults, the middle aged, and the elderly.[24] By obvious implication, an optimistic explanatory style is associated with positive emotional states, like happiness and joy.

This strong association is important because of studies that have linked increased depression with increased morbidity and mortality. These relationships hold above and beyond any influence of suicide, an all too common concomitant of severe depression. Indeed, the same pathways described in the previous section are implicated in the relationship between depression and immunosuppression.[25]

Depression Among our most common problems in the late twentieth century are disturbances in mood. Depression appears to be on the increase in contemporary society, which may seem ironic given the growing concern about feeling good.

There are two major types of mood disorder. In *depressive disorder,* the person experiences excessive unhappiness and despair. In *bipolar disorder* (formally called manic-depression), periods of inappropriate sadness (depression) alternate with periods of inappropriate elation (mania). There are cases of pure elation, but they are rare.

Continuity between normality and abnormality is nowhere better illustrated than in the case of depression, which refers to a transient mood—a person's appropriate reaction to disappointment—as well as to a chronic disorder. Where do we draw the line between normal depression and abnormal depression? Probably in no particular place. There are a number of signs and symptoms of depression, and the more present, the more severe the disorder.

Here are the ways in which people show depression:[26]

- depressed mood (which can be expressed as feeling sad, down, blue, in the dumps, empty, or irritable)
- loss of interest in pleasurable activities
- significant increase *or* decrease in appetite, resulting in weight gain or loss
- increase *or* decrease in sleep
- increase *or* decrease in physical activity, resulting in feelings of restlessness or sluggishness
- fatigue
- self-reproach: a belief that one is worthless, wicked, or stupid
- diminished ability to concentrate or make decisions
- thoughts of death and suicide; suicide plans; suicide attempts

Suicide as a depressive symptom deserves special mention. Although not all suicidal people are depressed, and not all depressed people are suicidal, the link between depression and suicide in our country is a strong one. Of the more than 200,000 known suicide attempts each year in the United States, perhaps 80% are carried out by seriously depressed individuals. So, depression is potentially a lethal disorder that should be taken seriously.

Consider these epidemiological facts about depression. First, one's lifetime chance of becoming depressed enough to warrant a diagnosis and clinical intervention is now estimated at somewhere between 8% and 23%. The frequency of depression has led to it being dubbed the common cold of psychopathology.[27] Second, depression occurs much more frequently among women than men, at least twice as much and perhaps eight times as much. Numerous explanations of this sex difference have been proposed implicating biological, psychological, and sociological factors, but none seems fully adequate at present.[28] Perhaps an explanation that integrates these different possibilities would resolve the puzzle about sex differences in depression. Third, the prevalence of depression among adults is largely independent of social class and race. Fourth, the *younger* the adult, the more likely he or she is to be depressed.

Let us take a look at the role of physiological processes in depression. What is the evidence that biology plays a role? To begin with, family studies show that if someone has a biological relative who is depressed, his or her chance of being depressed greatly increases. A comparable increase does not occur if one has an adoptive relative who is depressed. Also, the range of bodily symptoms in depression implies that the disorder is biological, because these symptoms fall into pairs, as we would expect if one's physical system were somehow out of balance: agitation *or* lethargy; too much sleep *or* too little; weight loss *or* weight gain. Another bit of support for a biological role in depression is that some physical illnesses (like thyroid disease) have depression as a consequence. Similarly, some medications produce depression as a side effect. And finally, depression can be successfully treated by a variety of biological interventions: drugs, electroconvulsive shock, and aerobic exercise.

Biological theories of depression posit low levels of neurotransmitters, particularly norepinephrine and serotonin, as the cause of the disorder. According to these theories, interventions succeed to the degree that they increase the level of these neurotransmitters. As it stands, our research methods are not sophisticated enough to measure norepinephrine and serotonin directly in the brains of depressed individuals, but the indirect evidence is strong. However, biological theories do not tell the whole story of depression. Recent years have seen the development of several psychological theories of depression that stress the role played by a person's cognitions. They propose that depression is predisposed and maintained by negative ways of thinking—by pessimism.

A cognitive theory of depression   Aaron Beck's cognitive theory,[29] presented in a popular way in the best seller *Feeling Good* by David Burns,[30] is one leading psychological account. Beck contends that depression is not so much a disorder of mood as one of thought. According to him, the depressed person thinks about herself, her world, and her future in pessimistic terms. Everything is bleak and grim. Presumably, she sees things as worse than they are. Why does she maintain this world view? Why don't events to the contrary challenge her depressive beliefs? Beck suggests two answers.

First, the depressed person is prone to *automatic thoughts:* unbidden and habitual ways of thinking that continually put her down. Suppose you are at a party, and you see an attractive person that you met a few weeks before. You might walk across the room to strike up a conversation. Then again, automatic thoughts might freeze you midstep:

> He won't remember who I am.
> He's probably waiting for his girlfriend.
> I'll say something stupid.

I have too much mousse in my hair.
It makes me look like Billy Idol.
I have nothing to say to him anyway.
I should have known—he's ignoring me already.
I hate parties.
I'm the only one not having fun.

And as though automatic thoughts like these were not depressing enough, Beck argues that depression is further maintained by errors in logic: slipshod ways of thinking that keep one's self-deprecating beliefs immune to reality. For instance, a depressed person selectively attends to bad events while overlooking good ones. On the way to pick up her Nobel Prize, let us suppose, someone gets a speeding ticket, and the ticket is all that she can think about for the rest of the week.

Or a depressed person may overly personalize the petty hassles of her everyday life. Waiting in a slow checkout line at the grocery store is proof positive that *she* is a loser, for picking this time to go shopping, for choosing that particular line, for believing that express checkout really means express, for living and breathing and needing to eat.

Beck's cognitive theory is influential because it accurately captures the way depressed people think and because it gives rise to an effective treatment of depression: cognitive therapy. In this approach, the therapist works with the depressed client to challenge her negative beliefs. These must first be made explicit, because automatic thoughts can be so ingrained that she pays little attention to them, only to their depressing consequences. Once on center stage, she can compare her automatic thoughts against the evidence and presumably find little justification for them.

Not that many decades ago, the outlook for depression was as bleak as the disorder itself. Little could be done for the depressive except to keep her from killing herself until her depression passed, usually (but not always) in three to six months. But now there is good news. Many successful treatments exist: antidepressant medication, social skills training, and talking therapies—notably Beck's approach. In Chapter 7, we will describe how an individual wishing to change his or her habitual thinking from pessimistic to optimistic can do so, using Beck's cognitive therapy techniques.

Learned helplessness and depression   As mentioned earlier, shortly after the learned helplessness phenomenon was first discovered in animals, Martin Seligman was struck by the similarity between animals made helpless following experience with uncontrollable events and people who were depressed.[31] He proposed that learned helplessness was analogous to depression, and indeed, that it provided a simple and efficient way to learn about depression. Helplessness could be produced reliably in the laboratory, whereas quite obviously depression could not be. If learned helplessness could serve as a laboratory model[32] for depression, possible treatments or preventions could be tried out on the model. The promising ones could then be generalized to the actual cases of depression.

Thus, the helplessness model has been explored on two fronts: in animal studies and in human studies. Table 5–1 summarizes the parallels that have been established. These are numerous and striking. In

TABLE 5–1. Parallels between Learned Helplessness and Depression

	Learned Helplessness	Depression
Symptoms	passivity	passivity
	cognitive deficits	self-blame
	self-esteem loss	low self-esteem
	sadness, hostility, anxiety	sadness, hostility, anxiety
	loss of appetite	loss of appetite
	sleep disruption	sleep disruption
	norepinephrine and serotonin depletion	norepinephrine and serotonin depletion
Causes	learned belief in response-outcome independence	generalized belief that responding is ineffective
Treatments	change belief in response futility	cognitive therapy
	antidepressant medication	antidepressant medication
	electroconvulsive shock	electroconvulsive shock
	time	time
Risk factor	pessimism	pessimism

Adapted from *Abnormal Psychology,* Second Edition, by David L. Rosenhan and Martin E. P. Seligman (p. 342), by permission of W. W. Norton & Company, Inc. Copyright ©1989, 1984 by W. W. Norton & Company, Inc.

particular, note that pessimism is a risk factor for both depression and learned helplessness. Studies measuring one's explanatory style with the Attributional Style Questionnaire find that individuals who explain bad events in a pessimistic fashion are more likely on the one hand to develop learned helplessness in the wake of bad events and on the other hand to become depressed in the same circumstances. We are thus on firm ground linking pessimism to depression, not only empirically but also theoretically.

The comparison is not perfect. First, there is a problem with respect to suicidal ideation. Learned helplessness shows itself not as the wish or attempt to die, but simply as passivity. In research by Beck and his colleagues, "hopelessness" is one of the key factors that predict suicide,[33] so we know that pessimism has something to do with suicide, but not in a way that our analogy clarifies.

Second, there is a problem with respect to sex differences, and particularly how they are manifested across the lifespan. As we noted earlier in the book, there is no good evidence that optimistic or pessimistic explanatory style distinguishes between men and women. Yet women are anywhere from two times to eight times more likely to be depressed than men. Interestingly, among children—before puberty—depression is somewhat more likely among males than females. The sex difference flip-flops—notably—with the onset of puberty and stays that way through the rest of life. The sex difference in depression is itself a hotly debated and frequently investigated issue. But the point here is that the learned helplessness analogy sheds little light on it.

Third, there is a problem with respect to the distinctions made within types of depression by diagnosticians. These do not map neatly into the distinctions of learned helplessness. This may represent a fault with the classification scheme typically used to describe depression, or it may be a shortcoming of the helplessness model, which treats all depressions as pretty much the same, except insofar as people use different causal explanations.

Fourth and relatedly, the learned helplessness model is not very relevant to bipolar disorder, although this could be simply because of the lack of theoretical effort.[34] Bipolar disorder seems to be genetically predisposed, although only 60% of those individuals with the identified gene for the problem actually develop the disorder.[35] This means that there is plenty of room left for other factors to play a role. How might optimism and pessimism fit in here? Psychoanalytic theorists have typically regarded mania as a defense against pessimism, which means that pessimistic thinking may play a role in bipolar disorder as well as in depressive disorder.

Finally, although the learned helplessness phenomenon seems to be a good analogy for depression, so too does it appear to be a good analogy for other ills of the human condition that involve passivity and pessimism. In a sense, learned helplessness is too rich a concept. We have already noted the numerous applications of the learned helplessness model. Theorists have failed to grapple with why uncontrollable events and subjective feelings of helplessness seem to produce depression in one group of people, academic failure in a second, cancer in a third, and listless work performance in a fourth. Perhaps such bad outcomes occur to the same group of people, in which case the learned helplessness model remains useful in its present form. But if different groups of people tend to suffer different sorts of problems, then the model must be expanded to explain why this is so.

Pessimism and negative feelings   Pessimistic explanatory style has been linked not simply to depressive symptoms but also to anxiety disorders, to eating disorders, and to other emotional problems. Perhaps the most reasonable thing to say about learned helplessness in general and explanatory style in particular is that they lead to a variety of negative emotional states, what psychologists and psychiatrists call dysphoria: simply feeling bad.[36] Dysphoria may take the form of depression; it may take the form of anxiety, or guilt, or anger, or hostility. The particular mix of these bad feelings probably depends on a host of other factors.

But for the purpose of linking optimism with good health and pessimism with poor health, this less-than-perfect mapping of helplessness and hopelessness into depression is to be expected, because recent evidence suggests that depression is not *uniquely* linked to poor health either. After reviewing several hundred investigations, Friedman and Booth-Kewley offer this conclusion:

> There is strong evidence of a reliable association between illness and chronic psychological distress. Hence, treatment of medical patients by . . . psychologists seems prudent and worthwhile.[37]

Chronic psychological distress includes emotional states like anxiety, anger, hostility, and/or depression. Research shows these to be associated with illnesses such as heart disease, asthma, ulcers, and arthritis, but the association is a general one, not a set of specific links matching particular emotions with particular illnesses. We suggest that pessimism is the underlying factor that cuts across these negative feelings and creates their association with poor health.

Defensive pessimism   There is a phenomenon that deserves attention, because it is a special case in which "negative" thinking appears to be beneficial for the individual. This is the idea of defensive pessimism, introduced by psychologists Julie Norem and Nancy Cantor.[38] They started with the observation that some individuals with a very good track record in some domain of achievement, such as school or work, nevertheless express very minimal expectations for how they will do on a coming challenge:

- I'm sure I'll flunk the test.
- I'm sure I'll botch that job.
- I'll never get a promotion.

Then these people go on to do perfectly well at whatever it was that they thought they would fail. Contrast defensive pessimism with positive denial and healthy illusions as we discussed them in Chapter 1; defensive pessimism embodies the exact opposite premise.

We might be tempted to dismiss these findings as simply unusual, an exception to the overwhelming evidence that pessimistic thinking is bad for an individual, but we should not rush to this conclusion. There is an important lesson here about positive and negative thinking, and how they relate to our emotions.

Norem and Cantor regard defensive pessimism as a strategy, a way to curb anxiety that might otherwise get in the way of achievement. They conducted a study of college students that makes this point. They identified defensive pessimists by looking first only at those with previously good academic records. Then among this group, they found people who expressed negative expectations about how they would do. When these negative thinkers were compared to other students with the same track record, there was no difference—on average—in their eventual academic performances. However, within each group, there turned out to be considerable variation in their grades. So, in this group, "pessimistic" expectations did not map onto subsequent performance.

But in a more detailed study, they posed a laboratory task to the defensive pessimists as well as to a comparable group who did not express negative expectations. The researchers then talked to some of the subjects, both defensive pessimists and others, before the task, telling them that they were sure to do well.

The defensive pessimists who were *not* engaged in this conversation did well, as did the other subjects whether or not they were talked to. But the defensive pessimists who were told that they would do well did not! What seemed to be a pep talk really turned out to be a detriment, because it distracted the defensive pessimists from using their negative statements to curb their anxiety.

Apparently the defensive pessimist takes pains to hold expectations in check when positive expectations might lead to disruptive anxiety. But remember that "pessimism" here is of a very special sort, and it proves useful only for those people with a good track record. Long-term follow-up studies by Norem and Cantor suggest that defensive pessimists eventually do hurt themselves, and their academic performance suffers. It seems as if their negative statements eventually take a toll on how well they do in school, and once again, we see that pessimism is harmful. We suspect that at least part of the problem incurred by defensive pessimists results when they voice their strategy to others. It is boring if not irritating to hear a successful individual talk about how poorly he or she will do. Eventually, people become turned off by what looks like fishing for a compliment.

What is the pertinence of defensive pessimism to the general relationship between optimism and health? In small doses, it is probably useful simply because it decreases negative emotions. As a way of life, it may not be good, because it will create a self-fulfilling prophecy.

Conclusions

In light of this discussion, let us look back at the questions raised but unanswered in Chapter 2. First, do optimism and pessimism affect the onset of a person's illness, or the course once it begins, or both? Granted the multiplicity of physiological and emotional consequences of these styles of thinking, we strongly suspect the answer is both. At the same time, optimism and pessimism do not operate in isolation from all the other possible influences on our bodies and our feelings. Someone in the pink of physical health will not court illness by an occasional negative thought. And someone at death's door will not be rescued by optimism.

Second, are optimism and pessimism related to particular types of illness—like cancer or heart disease—or to illness in general? Again, granted the multiplicity of consequences, we suspect that pessimism is a nonspecific risk factor and optimism a generic buffer.

There may be some intriguing exceptions, though. Allergies represent an overly sensitive immune system. We predict, therefore, that pessimism is associated with an absence of allergies. And we also predict that pessimists are good risks—in a biological sense, at least—for organ transplants, because their immune systems are less likely to reject foreign tissue.

Third, which criteria of poor health are most sensitive to optimism or pessimism? Probably those that rely on the individual's self-report of symptoms, although there are some subtleties involved in our logic. On the one hand, the individual is in a privileged position to know how he feels. Self-reports in principle can be more sensitive than "objective" medical tests. On the other hand, the individual is also subject to the tendency to distort how he feels, either for better or for worse. Optimism and pessimism might in turn affect these tendencies. Costa and McCrae, for instance, argue that "neurotic" individuals—who would be included among our dysphoric pessimists—exaggerate their symptoms.[39] Presumably, optimists do not.

In the short run, then, we have reason to distrust self-reported symptoms. But in the long run, we expect them to be valid, because they can set into operation the physiological and emotional processes we have described here. Even if the pessimist is not quite correct when he first describes his symptoms, he eventually will be.

Several intriguing studies by epidemiologists make a similar point.[40] When people are asked to rate their overall health—excellent, good, fair, or poor—at one point in time, this rating ends up predicting how long they live. Here is the punch line: "perceived" health translates itself into longevity even when every other factor that epidemiologists can think of is held constant statistically: sex, age, so-called objective health status as indexed by chronic diseases and disabilities, health practices, income, education, and so on. When those who considered their health "excellent" were compared to those who considered their health "poor," their risk of death within the subsequent decade was about one third.

One might think that perception of health is dictated by the facts of the matter, but this is not always the case. In an informal study, we talked to 18 of our friends about their medical history and how they currently perceived their health. We were struck by the independence of someone's perceptions of health and his or her actual illnesses. For instance, one individual has had high blood pressure for years and has suffered several serious heart attacks. He has severe arthritis in his hips and knees. How does he see his health? Without hesitation, at age

71, he told us that his current health is good, and he expects it to be even better in the future. In contrast, other individuals to whom we talked expressed a gloomy view of their health, even in the absence of past or present illnesses.

Finally, we asked about sex differences in the relationship of optimism and health. Here we tentatively conclude that optimism and pessimism do not explain the sex differences in morbidity and mortality. Although women are more likely than men to be depressed, and thus more likely to experience the sorts of illnesses that are made more likely by depression, we have no good evidence that the sex difference in depression originates in any tendency for women to be pessimistic and men to be optimistic. Indeed, our measures of explanatory style almost always yield the same average scores for men and women in our samples.

Our focus in the present chapter was on "internal" routes—those inside the person. We looked in particular at physiological and emotional paths. We turn in the next chapter to other routes, those that lie outside people and can therefore be more readily seen. Again, no single route is likely to constitute the sole link between optimism and health.

CHAPTER

6

From Optimism to Health: Behavioral and Interpersonal Routes

> Prayer indeed is good, but while calling on the gods a man should lend himself a hand.
>
> —*Hippocrates*

In this chapter, we continue surveying the routes between optimism and health, focusing on those that begin within the person (cognition) and find their destination there as well (health), but in between loop through the person's reciprocal relationship with the world. One of the most important of these is behavioral. Optimists act in different ways than do pessimists. For instance, many studies show that pessimists are poor problem solvers. They do not make good use of the evidence presented to them that things are better than they seem. And other studies show that the optimist perseveres when it is reasonable to do so, staying at a task until it is done. In contrast, the pessimist gives up and gives out. These characteristics of the optimistic person help him to achieve good health, whereas the characteristics of the pessimistic person may lead to ill health and even his early death.

111

Optimism and Problem Solving

Pessimists exemplify what psychologists refer to as the neurotic paradox: the tendency to make matters worse, to create many problems out of a few, never to leave bad enough alone. This tendency is a paradox given the assumption that people are ultimately hedonists, trying to maximize good feelings while minimizing bad ones. Why would anyone do things that create pain and misery?

Consider a recently overheard conversation:

"How are you doing?"

"Well, I'm not too happy. Fred asked me for a date again."

"And you don't want to see him."

"Exactly."

"So you turned him down?"

"No . . . I said to call me back later."

"And?"

"Well, I've been leaving my phone off the hook."

"But what about those job applications you've made? How can anyone reach you on the phone?"

"That's a problem."

No, that is two problems. Problem one is what to do about Fred. Problem two is what to do about being unemployed. And there may be a third and fourth problem lurking there as well.

Why do people behave this way? We do not find it paradoxical. Nor do we need to introduce a death wish as psychoanalytic theorists do. Rather, we see this tendency to make things worse as a consequence of certain ways of thinking, or to be more exact, certain ways of *not* thinking clearly about matters. The pessimist tends to think in precisely these unproductive ways, whereas the optimist thinks in more useful ways.

Let us examine several studies in detail that look at problem solving by optimists versus pessimists. A representative investigation is that of Alloy, Peterson, Abramson, and Seligman.[1] College students were recruited to participate in the experiment. Their first task was to complete the Attributional Style Questionnaire, so we could divide them into groups of optimists and pessimists, based on their scores.

Then we gave them a series of problems to solve. Each subject put on a pair of earphones and sat in front of a small box with two lights and three buttons on its top. A burst of white noise was delivered through the earphones, unpleasant but not harmful. The noise lasted five seconds unless the subject terminated it by pressing one of the buttons on the box. The lights indicated to the subject whether the noise had been successfully shut off within the time limit. This procedure was repeated, in all fifty times, with bursts of noise coming on every ten to thirty seconds.

As we discussed in Chapter 5, researchers interested in learned helplessness often induce helplessness in people by giving them tasks like this, and arranging matters so that they have no solution. Nothing that the research subject does will ever turn off the noise. A typical subject who works at unsolvable problems like these and then is given new problems to solve that indeed have solutions does not do particularly well. This is what we mean by helplessness.

But in the study described here there were some wrinkles. First, we knew who was an optimist and who was a pessimist, so we could compare their reactions to the uncontrollable noise. Second, when we moved from the initial phase of the study to the next phase, we used two different types of test problems. One type was highly similar to those in the initial phase, in other words, a series of loud noises delivered through headphones that research participants had to figure out how to turn off. The other type was highly dissimilar, in this case, scrambled words—jumbles or anagrams—that called on a subject to rearrange letters until they spelled a word.

Consistent with learned helplessness ideas, all subjects—optimists and pessimists alike—showed an impairment in problem solving when the test task was similar. They responded more slowly, they turned off the noise fewer times, and they took more trials to catch on to what was happening. We knew this would happen.

The more interesting comparison is with respect to the dissimilar problems. Here the pessimists again showed an impairment, solving the anagram problems poorly, slowly, or not at all. But the optimists showed no difficulty at all. They did just as well as subjects who never had the initial experience of helplessness. In short, they did not generalize their failure.

These results have some important implications for what we know about pessimism and optimism. They show that pessimists respond poorly to failure, generalizing their helplessness from one situation to a different one. Everyone will experience disappointments and setbacks in one domain of life or another. But pessimists take their dismay with them from this domain into others, where heretofore things may have gone well. In other words, pessimists make problems for themselves.

In contrast, optimists respond well to failure, shaking off the effects of a setback in one domain before they move on to another. Note that the optimists in our study were not oblivious to what happened in the initial phase of the experiment. They took a "helplessness" lesson with them to the second phase, when it was similar to the first. As W. C. Fields once said, "If at first you don't succeed, try again. Then quit. There's no sense being stupid about it."

Optimism should not be equated with mindless perseverance. But the optimist does not use failure in one sphere of life as a sign of impending failure in another. Perhaps she can be the best anagram solver who ever lived, regardless of how she did at pushing buttons to turn off noise. The problems of pessimists come in clumps, the problems of optimists singly.

Similar investigations of problem solving by optimists and pessimists among children have been carried out by psychologist Carol Dweck and her colleagues.[2] She studied grade school students, and her findings contain further lessons about optimism and pessimism. Dweck did not administer the Attributional Style Questionnaire to her research subjects. Instead, she used a related measure of the degree to which the children blamed themselves or not for academic failures. This is close to what we mean by pessimism versus optimism.

Then she presented these children with what are called discrimination problems, which give would-be solvers the task of discovering the principle used to designate certain abstract stimuli "correct" ones and others "incorrect" ones.

Imagine a formalized game of twenty questions. The experimenter shows the subject a big red square. He hazards a guess. "Yes, that's an example of what you are looking for." "Incorrect," says the experimenter. Then he is shown a medium yellow square. "Yes, that's an example." "Correct." Depending on the difficulty of the problem, finding a solution takes the subject anywhere from a few trials to many. But subjects eventually catch on and begin to abstract the rule that determines correct and incorrect feedback. Then they can discriminate readily among subsequent stimuli.

As we might expect, Dweck found that the optimistic children outperformed the pessimistic children. But what makes her studies particularly interesting was the children's approach to the problems. The optimistic children regarded them as challenges. They were eager for the next one. If a problem did prove too difficult for them, they enjoyed it all the more. In contrast, the pessimistic children moped and sulked. They did not want to work on the problems, particularly difficult ones. They failed to persevere. They interpreted every failure as a sign of their incompetence. And they made irrelevant comments.

Psychologists refer to what the optimistic and pessimistic children were variously doing as "framing" the problems they encountered. A concept identification problem can be depicted as a disaster waiting to happen or as a challenge. A recent television show described the World Series of 1975 between the Cincinnati Reds and the Boston Red Sox. Game Six has been described as the greatest baseball game ever played. Boston won at the very end of the game on a dramatic home run by Carlton Fisk.

According to the television show, Pete Rose—then a player for Cincinnati—enthused to Cincinnati manager Sparky Anderson after the game, saying in effect, "That was the best game I've ever played in." Anderson was dumbstruck. "Pete, we lost the game." "So what," was Rose's response. "We'll beat 'em the next time. But wasn't that a great game!"

During the 1989 baseball season, Pete Rose was banned from baseball for gambling. But we assume that he will make a comeback from his darkest hour. And what about Sparky Anderson, who could not make sense of Rose's enthusiasm in the wake of defeat? In 1989, he was the Detroit manager; he took a leave from his team because of what was described as exhaustion but also sounded a lot like demoralization. His team finished with a dismal record. An interview with Sparky in *The Sporting News* confirms our analysis of him as someone who frames setbacks poorly:

> I don't believe there's ever been an individual . . . who takes losses harder and keeps them inside longer than I do. I won't kid you, I was mentally exhausted. I could not have gone one more day. I had taken it so hard that it worked my body up to the point my hand was shaking. I've always told young players that nothing is so important in baseball that it should ruin your life. The sun will always shine tomorrow. I've always talked those words, but I've never listened to them. . . . At this stage in my career, I don't believe I can hold every loss inside. The chemicals inside of the body won't allow it, and when the body fires back at you, it fires hard.[3]

It is clear that the way people frame the problems and tasks of life is critical to how they approach them. Sometimes a problem eludes a solution, but it can still be regarded as a learning experience.

Optimists are more willing and more able to do this than pessimists, who take each and every failure to heart and assume that the future will be just like the present.

Optimism and Achievement

Let us now move to another sphere of problem solving—academic achievement. Not everyone may be convinced that studies of abstract shapes and scrambled words allow for good generalizations about life outside the laboratory. But studies of how optimistic and pessimistic students fare in their coursework surely can be generalized to real life. Indeed, to tens of millions of people in the United States, school *is* real life, because they are currently enrolled in courses. Virtually all Americans have attended or will attend school at some point in their life.

College students   In a series of studies, we looked at how college students who have completed the ASQ do in their schoolwork. In one investigation, Peterson and Barrett asked 87 entering freshmen at Virginia Tech to complete a version of the ASQ just as the school year began.[4] These students then gave us permission to check their academic records at the end of the school year, which we did. We ascertained their grade point averages, and discovered a moderate correlation between optimism and doing well.

Comparing the grades of those in the most pessimistic 25% of the sample with those in the most optimistic 25%, we found that the grades of the former group averaged just below a C, and those of the latter group averaged close to B−. These are meaningful differences at most universities. Students with B− averages or better often can elect certain options like pass-fail courses not otherwise available. Persons with grade point averages below C are usually on probation, and athletes may be prohibited from participation in sports. Students and athletes alike could lose scholarships. And they may not graduate if their grades stay at this level.

We also knew the Scholastic Aptitude Test (SAT) scores for our subjects. These test scores are required for admission at most colleges and universities. Despite controversies surrounding the SAT, its scores continue to be used because they bear a moderate to strong relationship with the grades achieved in college. In other words, all things being equal, students with higher SAT scores do better than students with lower SAT scores. So how does our measure of optimism and pessimism fare with respect to the ability of the SAT to predict the grades of these students?

First, the relationship between optimism and grades is not quite so robust as the relationship between SAT scores and grades—but it is in the ballpark. Second, the ASQ predicts grades independently of the SAT. They are not redundant. It is popular in some quarters to interpret SAT scores as an index of intelligence. Others strongly disagree. Regardless, everyone thinks it would be desirable to find a way of predicting success in school that does not depend just on the sorts of skills that the SAT taps. Perhaps measuring optimism is a candidate for this alternative way of predicting academic success.

In another study, this one done with University of Michigan students, we took a look at the study habits of optimistic and pessimistic students.[5] Our findings suggest why optimists might be better students than pessimists. In contrast to pessimists, here is how optimistic students approach studying and learning. In response to a questionnaire, they reported that they:

- set their own goals for themselves
- do *not* rely on externally imposed goals
- perceive themselves as competent
- do *not* experience anxiety during examinations
- employ various strategies for learning material—like rehearsal and imposing an organization
- take a broad view of their own learning, showing skill at what psychologists call *metacognition*—thinking about thinking—and hence can plan, monitor, and regulate their own problem solving
- think critically
- think originally
- manage the setting in which they study
- seek help from others when needed

Is it any surprise that optimists do better at their school work than pessimists? Again these relationships occur above and beyond SAT scores. These are not simply things that conventionally "intelligent" people do. Optimism and pessimism as we construe them cut across typical designations of intelligence.[6]

Note the theme of "framing" that runs through the learning skills of optimistic students. When given a problem set or an essay or an exam question, they do not simply sit there hoping the finished product appears. Rather, they arrange things—both internally and externally—so that a good solution to the task at hand is more likely to occur. They become captains of their own ship, and not surprisingly, they seldom run aground.

Harness racing patrons   The fraction of a percent of Americans who have never set foot in a school may be hanging out in pool halls or at racetracks. We have no data on pool halls, but a study we did at a racetrack showed that optimism and pessimism affect the achievement that takes place there as well (by those who place bets, not by the horses).

For most patrons at the track, the goal of betting is to win some money. Atlas and Peterson visited a harness racing track in central Michigan on two occasions.[7] With permission from the powers that be, we set up a table and placed a large sign there requesting participants for a psychology experiment on decision making. We promised to pay each subject ten dollars for completing a few questions before the race, and then a race-by-race diary about their bets: how much they wagered on a given race, whether they won or lost, and whether they were ruminating about previous and future races while they should have been thinking about the race at hand.

In all, 53 individuals participated—31 men and 22 women— with an average age of 43. They seemed to be serious bettors, coming to a harness racetrack about 39 times a year, each time bringing about $80 to bet for the day. The typical participant also reported breaking even or coming out ahead on most days at the track. We have a few doubts about the veracity of this information, although we are willing to accept the other data provided by these bettors.

We collected the questionnaires and the race-by-race diaries and paid the subjects their money. Clever researchers that we were, we stopped the study with a few races to go, to allow any of our subjects who were tapped out to place one last bet. This made the study highly attractive to prospective subjects as well as to the track officials.

When a bet was lost on a given race, which happened to the majority of the subjects the majority of the time, individuals rated as pessimistic on the ASQ ruminated more about other races than did optimists. We assume that the optimists were instead planning their next bets. The more bettors ruminated, the worse their subsequent betting became.

Although we neglected to ascertain the odds of each wager, the pattern of results implies that pessimism leads to increasingly large wagers with ever more remote odds. This does not work out for the bettor, and we suspect that a vicious circle is thereby entered. More losses lead to more rumination, more rumination leads to worse bets, worse bets lead to more losses.

We do not know if any of these subjects had a problem with gambling. But a study by Richard McCormick and Julian Taber shows that compulsive gamblers score in the pessimistic direction on the Attributional Style Questionnaire, attributing bad events in their lives to internal, stable, and global causes.[8] And the more severe their gambling problems, the more pessimistic they are.

This depiction of the compulsive gambler as a pessimist is interesting.[9] Surely one might think that a gambler is an optimist. Why bet in light of negative expectations for the future? But remember how we characterized optimism and pessimism in Chapter 1. Optimism is grounded in reality. An optimist, as a realist, knows in the first place that *all* bets favor the house. We suspect that truly optimistic people do not gamble at all, or if they do gamble, it is for fun and not profit. An optimist who does bet will make a wise bet, not a dumb one, and—on the average—long shots are particularly dumb bets. That is why they are called long shots.

A pessimist would favor long shots, as we see it, because the only perceived way to get ahead in the world is to throw oneself on the winds of chance and see where they blow. Once in a while this will pay off, which keeps the bettor hooked. Betting, whether on baseball games, harness races, the roulette wheel, or the lottery, may seem a preferable course to the individual who believes that his or her own actions amount to nothing in the world. We will see another example of this, perhaps more insidious, when we later describe the "safer sex" practices of gay men at high risk for AIDS.

Optimism and Goal Setting

Let us go back to school, to describe studies that looked at how optimistic versus pessimistic students set goals for themselves. Here is a place where these groups would be expected to differ, because optimism and pessimism of necessity involve expectations about the future. But the difference in the goals set by optimists and pessimists is not as simple as positive expectations on the one hand versus negative expectations on the other. Indeed, people rarely set "negative" goals for themselves.[10] The differences between the goals of an optimist and those of a pessimist are more subtle.

First, optimists set more *specific* goals for themselves than do pessimists.[11] An optimistic student might say that her goals for the coming school year are to achieve a B+ average, to secure a summer internship in her planned field, and to assist Professor Jones in assembling a bibliography on acid rain. A pessimistic student might say that his goals for the year are to learn a lot, to keep his options open, and to get to know some of his teachers better.

Perhaps these two sets of goals seem equally laudable. Perhaps the pessimistic student's goals even seem preferable because they sound grander yet at the same time more flexible. But research consistently shows that specific goals are associated with much better performance than general goals.[12] Psychologists who study goals and motivation even have a name for those vague goals that fail to translate themselves into successful performance: DYB goals, for "do your best" goals. Whether advising workers in industry or students in school, they counsel strongly against DYB goals. Our research shows that the optimist has figured this out already, without the advice of experts.

Another difference between the goals of optimists and pessimists lies not in the stated goal itself, but in the individual's *confidence* that it can be achieved. This is what Bandura calls self-efficacy,[13] as we explained in Chapter 3. A person's goals per se are not accomplished unless there is some motivation at work, and motivation is present only when that person is confident in his abilities to do what he has set out to do.

Cognitive approaches in psychology can be criticized for legitimizing a too "rational" view of people, one that renders them calm, cool, and collected while disregarding the importance of passion. This is a curious criticism, because it fails to reflect even a casual reading of the research literature. When we read about the effect of a person's thoughts on her behavior, we find her motives front and center in almost every discussion. Motivation reflects beliefs. Motives are *the* way that beliefs are translated into action.

To recapitulate, we have been arguing that optimists differ from pessimists in how they think. They are better problem solvers, in part because they can frame problems in better ways, in part because they set goals for themselves that are specific, and in part because they have the confidence that they can achieve their goals. We see an obvious tie-in here with health. Optimists, because they are better problem solvers than pessimists, end up with fewer problems in life. We saw in Chapter 3 that stressful life events as well as everyday hassles take a toll on one's well-being. We suspect that optimists have fewer major life events as well as fewer mundane problems, because they take a proactive approach to the challenges of life, anticipating and heading off difficulties as much as possible, defusing or minimizing them otherwise.

Even when optimists and pessimists confront the same problems in life, the optimists often fare better because they persevere. A series of studies has documented the stick-to-it-iveness of optimists. We include here studies that look in particular at health-promoting activities. Optimists are healthier than pessimists in part because they work harder at being healthy. At least part of the link between optimism and health is that simple.

Optimism and Perseverance

Optimistic thinkers bounce back particularly well from setbacks. Consider a study by Martin Seligman and Peter Schulman, who administered the ASQ to 101 insurance agents who were just beginning their careers.[14] Selling insurance is an occupation fraught with setbacks and disappointments. The agent must make numerous contacts before a single appointment can be arranged. Numerous appointments must take place before a single policy can be sold. If there were ever a career that required someone to be good at shaking off the effects of failure, it is selling insurance.

Thinking along these lines, Seligman and Schulman expected that an agent's characteristic optimism or pessimism would predict the course of his or her career. This is exactly what they found. They looked at who resigned from their jobs within twelve months of their initial training. Only 42 agents out of the original 101 were still with the company after the first year, and optimists were twice as likely to have survived as pessimists. For those agents among the most optimistic quarter of the sample, the dropout rate was about 30%, and for those among the most pessimistic quarter, the dropout rate was about 70%.

Seligman and Schulman also looked at the performance of those who stayed with the job for twelve months. They found that the optimistic salespeople sold more policies than the pessimistic ones, and that these totaled more money. Again, we see a link between optimism and perseverance, one that probably holds in a variety of jobs that place a premium on perseverance.

One more example from school shows how optimism translates itself into perseverance. Peterson, Colvin, and Lin administered the ASQ to 40 summer school students at the University of Michigan at the beginning of the term.[15] Each research participant kept a weekly log of successes and failures in the course being taken, and each noted any attempts he or she made to bolster performance in the wake of failure—getting extra help from the instructor, hiring a tutor, consulting a supplementary textbook in the library, and so on. We again found an association between optimism and perseverance. Optimistic students, following a failure, initiated more active attempts to improve their grades than did pessimistic students.

Still another example: Minou Alexander studied 56 caretakers of severely head-injured individuals.[16] How do these people—usually parents or spouses—handle the myriad of cognitive and interpersonal difficulties created by a head injury to a loved one? Those with such injuries may show profound personality changes. They might become extremely forgetful. They might be rigid in their thinking. And they might be impulsive or emotional. This is not easy to cope with. Some caretakers become passive and despondent, yet others go about their business perfectly well. An interesting and consistent finding from the research literature is that objective indices of brain damage bear no particular relationship to the burden the caretaker experiences. Accordingly, the psychological characteristics of the caretaker warrant special attention, and optimism versus pessimism is an apt characteristic for study.

Alexander administered the ASQ to the caretakers in her sample and found that optimists reported a better mood and more active coping attempts than those with a pessimistic view of bad events. Again, a clear pathway between optimism and perseverance is established, even when a measure of "objective" brain damage (i.e., the length of time the individual was unconscious immediately following the injury) was held constant statistically.

Martin Seligman, Susan Nolen-Hoeksema, Nort Thornton, and Karen Moe Thornton conducted yet another study of optimism and perseverance in the face of setbacks.[17] Their subjects were 33 varsity swimmers, 14 men and 19 women, at a well-known West Coast university. All athletes completed the ASQ. Then the swimming coaches had each subject swim a timed race in his or her best event. In each case, a false time was given to the swimmer, one considerably slower than what he or she had actually achieved. Following this feedback, the swimmer then swam a second timed race.

As we would expect, their habitual levels of optimism or pessimism predicted how the swimmers performed during the second race relative to the first race. Although both optimists and pessimists believed they had performed badly in the first race, the optimistic swimmers improved their performance, whereas the pessimistic swimmers did worse.

In sum, diverse studies, with insurance agents, college students, caretakers of head-injured relatives, and varsity swimmers, show that optimism is associated with perseverance, particularly in the face of disappointments and setbacks. This suggests that optimists also persevere in the sphere of health promotion. We predict that optimists are more likely to follow a healthful lifestyle and more likely to muster their resources in the face of illness.

Optimism and Health Promotion

Those with a pessimistic view of the causes of events act helplessly, suggesting that one route from pessimism to poor health is passivity in health care. Several studies support this extrapolation.

Healthful habits   For instance, Peterson assessed the explanatory style of 126 college students,[18] along with their reported adherence to habits identified by epidemiologists as associated with good health and a long life[19]:

- eating a balanced diet
- avoiding salt
- avoiding fat
- exercising
- eating breakfast
- not smoking
- not drinking to excess
- sleeping eight hours a night

Pessimistic subjects were less likely than optimistic subjects to engage in these health-promoting activities.

In learned helplessness terms, the pessimists are taking the easy way out. This conclusion is buttressed by confidence ratings made by these subjects concerning whether they believed they could change their bad health habits. Pessimists expressed less confidence that they would or could change. This finding is particularly important in light of reports that most people who break their bad health habits try several times before they succeed. For instance, among those who quit smoking, it takes an average of three relapses before the habit is finally broken.[20]

Responses to illness   Another study of optimism and health-related behaviors was carried out by Peterson, Colvin, and Lin.[21] Seventy-two young adults in Ann Arbor first completed the ASQ and then for several weeks kept track of symptoms of illness they experienced as well as what—if anything—they did in order to feel better. Optimistic individuals were *less likely* to fall ill than pessimists, but when they did become ill, they were *more likely* to take active steps to feel better—resting more, increasing their intake of fluids, and the like.

Let us detail another finding from this investigation. Suppose a person was sick during one week and took active steps to feel better. Did this mean he was less likely to be sick the next week? The answer is no. Doing active things had no demonstrable effect on the course of one's illness. This finding was at first a bit surprising and a little disappointing. It seems to be inconsistent with the story we have been telling. But then we realized that we were expecting effects of "healthy" habits to take place on a time scale that was implausible.

Indeed, if simply resting one week made illness less likely the following week, this obvious relationship could be discerned by anyone—optimists and pessimists alike. Society would not spend so many resources mounting health promotion campaigns if the connection between behavior and good health were direct and immediate, as opposed to subtle and distant. The very nature of these relationships is that they are nonobvious and take years or even decades to unfold. After all, public service announcements do not caution citizens against gargling with lye or sticking their hands in fans—behaviors that will have an immediate effect on one's well-being.

We know that links exist between behavior and health; epidemiological evidence is unambiguous in documenting the relationships between certain habits and one's long-term health status. For instance, people who smoke live on the average eight years less than those who do not smoke. So why do people smoke? Because the eight years come off of the far end of life. If everyone who lit up a cigarette

suddenly lost the next eight years, the Surgeon General's warning on cigarette packages would be unnecessary. Nobody would smoke. Nobody.

The point is that a person's inclination to act on documented links between her behavior and subsequent health must be based on her belief. She must expect with confidence that what she does or does not do today will have effects, for better or for worse, in the distant future. This is exactly what optimism entails, of course, and so our results do make sense. Optimists take preventive steps when they are ill, even though the payoffs are not immediate. Indeed, the benefits of health promotion are not even guaranteed. They are simply generalizations. But as we have been trying to stress throughout the book, the optimist goes with what is likely. What other realistic choice is there?

In our next study that looked at the association between explanatory style and health-related behavior, Lin and Peterson administered the ASQ to 96 University of Michigan students, along with a questionnaire describing various active responses to illness[22] (see Table 6–1). Respondents were asked what they usually did when they fell ill in order to feel better. Optimistic individuals were more likely

TABLE 6–1. *Active Responses to Illness*

I increase my rest and sleep.
I am more likely to go to bed on time.
I cut back on strenuous exercise.
I decrease my work load.
I visit a doctor or a clinic.
I take over-the-counter medication.
I take prescription medication.
I increase vitamins.
I eat more nutritious food than usual.
I eat less junk food than usual.
I am more likely to eat meals on schedule.
I increase my fluids (juice, soup, and so on).
I get more fresh air than usual.
I get more sunlight than usual.
I use a humidifier.
I use extra covers on my bed.
I increase the temperature in my room.
I put aside any worries I might have.

---

to take active steps—individually and collectively—than were pessimistic individuals.

The same subjects were also asked to describe their most recent
bout of illness, as well as their reaction to this episode, using the Ways
of Coping questionnaire devised by Lazarus and Folkman.[23] Part of
this questionnaire asks a respondent to describe what is at "stake"
during a stressful event. There was an association between pessimism
and an individual's fear that he or she would be rejected or ridiculed
for falling ill. We will return to this finding in the next section when
we talk about the interpersonal aspects of optimism and pessimism.
But for now the point is that the pessimist who falls ill seems to face
two problems—the illness itself and a fear of rejection by others because of the illness.

Also part of the Ways of Coping measure are particular coping
attempts that a person may or may not make in a specific situation.
We identified a number of responses that seemed to show either a
"helpless" reaction to illness or its opposite "active" reaction, like the
following:

- I blamed myself (helpless)
- I went along with fate (helpless)
- I felt bad because I couldn't avoid the situation (helpless)
- I realized I brought the problem on myself (helpless)
- I made a plan of action and followed it (active)
- I came up with a couple of different solutions (active)

A composite measure of these responses showed a moderately strong
relationship to a person's explanatory style. Optimists were active in
their attempts to cope with illness; pessimists were helpless.

Safer sex   We want to describe one more study of the relationship
between optimism and health-promoting behavior. This research
took us into eight Detroit area gay bars between December 1 and December 11, 1987. We were interested in the relationship between
someone's optimism and pessimism and whether he engaged in "safer
sex" practices in order to prevent the transmission of AIDS. These
particular bars variously catered to black or white customers, older or
younger, and the Yuppie crowd as well as the leather set.

In all, 96 homosexual and bisexual men completed several questionnaires, including a measure of optimism-pessimism[24] as well as a

standard questionnaire developed by Jennifer Bryce of the Michigan Department of Public Health that asked respondents about:

- knowledge of AIDS transmission routes
- knowledge of AIDS prevention strategies
- the "safer sex" practices they were or were not following
- perceived risk for AIDS

The results were clear-cut. There was no overall relationship between a subject's optimism and his knowledge of AIDS. In other words, both optimists and pessimists knew the same things about the transmission and prevention of AIDS. In fact, both groups knew a great deal. This is by now a typical finding in the United States. Almost everyone has taken in the widely publicized information about AIDS.

But despite the fact that everyone knew about AIDS—how it is spread and how it can be prevented—we did find differences among these men in whether they engaged in "safer sex" practices. The more pessimistic individuals were less likely to take such precautions as reducing the number of their sexual partners or using a condom during sexual activity. The more optimistic individuals did take these precautions.

If optimists were Pollyannas who expected that everything will turn out for the best, perhaps we would expect the optimists in our sample to take risks. Such was not the case, and once again our richer view of optimism is vindicated. We see optimism as a realistic belief that a person translates into appropriate action, as we saw among the men we studied in the gay bars of Detroit. If people expect to be around in the future, then they take steps to be sure that they will be. The more pessimistic subjects in our study saw themselves at greater risk for AIDS than did the optimistic ones. We assume that fatalism—that is, perceived independence between responses and outcomes—was operating among the pessimists. If someone expects to contract AIDS, then why bother to change how one behaves?

Health promotion   So, several studies have shown that optimism is reflected in behavior that aims at either preventing illness in the first place or minimizing its effects once it occurs. That someone's actions can provide a route between optimism and physical well-being is thus quite likely, suggesting a ready target for the health professional who wishes to intervene and help people lead longer and more satisfying lives.

How has health been promoted in the past? The health professions have gone through three major eras in their attempt to combat illness.[25] In the first era, responses were strictly reactive in nature. Once someone became ill, she received treatment. In the second era, attempts were made to prevent people from getting ill in the first place by modifying their physical environment, reducing the likelihood that they would become infected by germs. Swamps containing malaria-bearing mosquitoes were drained. Trash heaps housing rats that carried fleas that carried the bubonic plague were removed. Surgeons washed their hands before and after operations.

Both of these eras were important, and we obviously still deploy strategies from them today. But the third era of combating illness is far more sophisticated. At this point, it is estimated that most people die from illnesses that have something to do with their lifestyle. Smoking, drinking, poor nutrition, and lack of exercise contribute to an incredible number and variety of maladies. Indeed, it is estimated that at least half of all hospital admissions have something to do with people's behavior. So, in the third and most recent era of combating illness, we try to induce people to get rid of their unhealthy habits.

This era differs from the other two because no longer is the individual allowed to stand on the sidelines while physicians fight germs and public health workers alter the physical environment. He is required to act differently. Health promotion is not a spectator sport. To this end, an incredible number of programs have been undertaken—in the media, in schools, at work, and even in whole communities and nations—that try to encourage people to act in healthful ways.

Peterson and Stunkard recently reviewed the vast literature on health promotion.[26] Despite its promise, we came up with some disappointing conclusions. Health promotion is currently a field without a unifying theory of how to change people's behavior for the better. What it is in effect is a heap of techniques, some of which work some of the time, some of which work other times, and some of which never work—all with no good explanation why. The typical health promotion message is a mixture of simplistic moral exhortation and complex technical information. ("Let's see, is this 'good' cholesterol or 'bad' cholesterol?") Perhaps not surprisingly, some people—especially minorities and those in the lower-income groups—are notoriously unreached and thus unmoved by these messages.

One of the problems with current health promotion programs is that they treat all people the same, neglecting important social and personality differences. We think that health promotion programs should pay attention to someone's level of optimism or pessimism. The optimist and the pessimist need different messages. The optimist may merely need to be told the right information. The pessimist may need to have her sense of efficacy boosted before such information becomes relevant to her.

Optimism and Interpersonal Relations

We will now consider one final link between optimism and good health. We have mentioned several times already that other people have something to do with one's physical well-being. People with a rich network of supportive individuals to whom they can turn in trouble live longer and healthier lives. They are more robust in the face of stress and hassles in everyday life.[27] The existence of friendships is a good predictor of health and longevity.[28] Even people with pets seem to outlive people who do not have one to keep them company.[29] There is something healthful about a good companion, whether with two legs or four legs.

On the other hand, deficient or ruptured human relationships can take a toll on health and happiness. Remember the bereavement studies described in Chapter 3. In the six months following the death of a spouse, the surviving individual is at increased risk for death. People who are lonely do not live as long—in spite of the fact that they may not be coming into contact with as many germs as people with lots of friends.

It is not our purpose to explain all the effects of other people on someone's physical health. The influences of social support and social interaction on health are fully as complex as those of optimism, and they probably share many of the same pathways—physiological, emotional, and behavioral. Rather, let us just take these effects as a given, and spend the remainder of this chapter examining the relationship between optimism and getting along with others. The yield of this examination is the specification of yet another route between optimism and health—one that runs through good interpersonal relationships.

Loneliness   Craig Anderson and his colleagues have shown in several studies that pessimists are lonely and socially estranged.[30] They administered a version of the ASQ to research subjects along with a standard questionnaire measuring loneliness that asks how frequently they experience feelings like the following:

- There is no one I can turn to.
- I feel left out.
- No one really knows me well.
- My social relationships are superficial.

The link between pessimism and loneliness is as robust as that between pessimism and depression, prompting Anderson to suggest that these are not altogether separate phenomena. We concur. Optimists, of course, have more numerous and more satisfying social relationships.

Why are pessimists so lonely? A study by Gotlib and Beatty gives a clue.[31] They asked research subjects to read about hypothetical individuals who described their lives and what was happening in them. Everything was the same about the vignettes with the exception of the causal explanations that were tucked into the narratives. Some of the scenarios depicted people who were optimistic in their explanations, i.e., using external, unstable, and specific causes. Others depicted people who explained events in a pessimistic fashion with internal, stable, and global causes. Then Gotlib and Beatty asked for their responses to these people. Subjects rejected the pessimists and felt attracted to the optimists. Think about how we respond to someone who is pessimistic. We may want to cheer them up or give them hope, but their assertions that nothing can be done are daunting, to say the least.

It is certainly clear that depression and pessimism are contagious states. Depression runs through families. So too does pessimism. We have shown, for instance, that pessimistic parents also have pessimistic children.[32] Perhaps many people recognize this fact about pessimism, and take pains to protect themselves from the corrosive presence of a pessimistic acquaintance.

We do not believe that anyone has looked at this matter, but we speculate that pessimists—in addition to whatever other problems they may have—are notably deficient at fending off others who will rain on their already soggy parades. We suspect that they do not actively pursue friends, but rather take in whoever walks through the front door. They do not call the shots in their relationships. To the degree that the pessimist ends up with other pessimistic people as friends—and this seems to be what happens—we have yet another one of those vicious circles by now so familiar to us when we look at pessimism. The relevance to physical well-being is obvious. The pessimist does not receive the benefits of "other people." The optimist's cup runneth over, as usual.

Social consequences of pessimism   We conducted a recent study that clarifies the interpersonal nature of pessimism and optimism.[33] Originally, we were interested in what people in general mean by "helpless" behavior. We knew what psychologists mean by helplessness—the passivity and listlessness that uncontrollability produces in dogs and people. But what do people in general mean when they describe someone as helpless?

To this end, we used a procedure devised by psychologists David Buss and Kenneth Craik for making abstract psychological states concrete in terms of the behaviors that reflect them.[34] We asked a large number of college students to think of people they knew who were helpless. Then we asked them to describe the sorts of things these people did that showed their helplessness. We then requested another group of individuals to go through this list of several hundred possible behaviors and rate each for how good an example of helplessness it seemed to be. The very best examples were then identified and used to create a measure of general helplessness (see Table 6–2).

In the next phase of our research, 75 college students reported on the frequency with which they had performed each of these helpless behaviors during the past month. They also completed the ASQ. As expected, pessimism was associated with an increased frequency of performing helpless behaviors. Said another way, optimists did not act in these ways. We have some confidence in these results because a friend of each subject completed a questionnaire about the subject's helplessness, and these reports strongly validated those of the actual subjects.

A close look at Table 6–2 reveals that some of these very good examples of helplessness are interpersonal in nature. In other words, helpless individuals seem to involve others in their plight. This has intriguing implications, but it also raises the possibility that "helplessness" is not as ineffectual as it might seem. Perhaps acting in these ways is instrumental because it leads others to do the bidding of the individual who proclaims his or her own inability.

A follow-up study argues against this interpretation. College students at Michigan were asked to think of a particular friend, and then to report the frequency with which the friend performed the behaviors

TABLE 6–2. *Prototypically Helpless Behaviors*

I didn't leave my house / apartment all day.
I didn't cook for myself.
I was unable to fix a broken object.
I cried.
I gave up in the middle of doing something.
I said negative things about myself.
I didn't compete when given the opportunity.
I didn't study because "it doesn't matter."
I let someone take advantage of me.
I asked others to do something for me.
I didn't stand up for myself.
I didn't change a strategy that does not work.
I failed to make an important decision.
I stayed in an abusive relationship.
I let someone else make a decision for me.
I used another person as a crutch.
I refused to do something on my own.

---

in Table 6–2. Finally, subjects were asked to describe how *they* responded to the friend when he or she acted in these ways. Friends who only infrequently acted in a helpless fashion were given help and sympathy when they did. But if the friends frequently acted helplessly, they were treated with anger or ignored or avoided. Who could blame our subjects? Being around listless people takes a toll.

So, these results cohere, showing that pessimistic people are lonely and socially estranged from others . . . because they turn people off . . . because they act in excessively helpless ways.[35] In the short run, a friend can and does meet the needs and demands of someone who requires assistance. This is rewarding and the very business of friendship. But in the long run, most people do not continue to meet such demands. It must seem to them as if the pessimistic person is never satisfied—and that is the point. The friend of the pessimist can himself become pessimistic as he begins to feel "helpless" because of the lack of any connection between what he does and how his friend acts. Or he can pick up and leave. He will take the latter course more often than not, we suppose, leaving the pessimistic person without the buffer against ill health that good relationships can provide.

This cannot be entirely a mystery to the pessimist. Let us return to the finding we described earlier that a pessimistic person who falls ill fears that she will be rejected by others because of her illness. On the face of it, this seems like a groundless fear. By and large, people do not blame each other for falling ill, nor should they ever (remember our discussion of blaming the victims of illness in Chapter 2). But perhaps the pessimistic person is like the boy who cried wolf, complaining so frequently that others become indifferent to further requests for aid and support, now legitimate granted the person is ill. Here is another example of the pessimist making things worse than they need to be.

In this chapter and the previous one, we have discussed a number of the routes that can take someone from optimism to good health: physiological, emotional, behavioral, and interpersonal. Figure 6–1 presents an overview of these pathways. Here and there we have mentioned how one route intersects with another. Depression influences the immune system, for instance, and interpersonal relations influence depression. We have not drawn in all of these influences in Figure 6–1, because it would turn our nice diagram into a confusing tangle. Just appreciate the complexity that is involved in translating optimism into good health—or pessimism into poor health, for that matter.

Granted the multiplicity of these influences and their plausibility individually and collectively, it seems bizarre that some people still regard health as simply a matter of biological forces. In their reductionistic approach, the only "real" explanation is on the ostensibly basic level of biology. This strategy strikes us as wrong.

FIGURE 6–1.   The Routes Between Optimism and Health

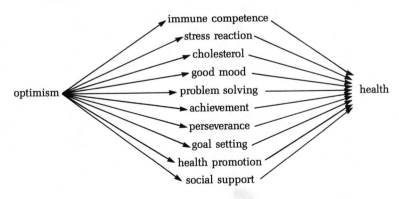

One important implication of this conclusion is that people can change in very basic ways by changing how they think. And if they think differently, perhaps they will become more healthy. We consider how to encourage people to become more optimistic in the following chapter.

CHAPTER

7

Becoming
an Optimist

We must live as we think, otherwise we shall end up thinking as
we have lived.

—*Paul Bourget*

Optimism and pessimism are highly
stable dispositions, but they can change in response to events throughout
our lives. Those who wish to become more optimistic should, obviously,
try to arrange matters so that events that encourage optimism are more
likely to occur and those that undercut it are less likely to occur.

As we emphasized earlier, however, mere exhortations to be positive do not set into motion long-lasting changes. People are unable to
embrace or discard complex beliefs simply because it would be healthful to do so. We believe as we do—whether optimistically or pessimis-
tically—because our styles of believing are ingrained. These styles
develop slowly, as a function of repeated experiences like those described in Chapter 4; the process of changing them must be ap-
proached with considerable patience.

The Web of Belief

We have described in detail the consequences of these styles of believing, in particular good and bad health. We have speculated about

135

their origins. And we have talked about the mechanisms via which optimism and pessimism are related to health status.

Self-evidently, optimistic and pessimistic beliefs do not exist in a vacuum. They are related to other beliefs, in belief *systems*. What is a belief system? The many beliefs that a person has—about himself, the world, the past, the present, and the future, the price of tea and/or democracy in China—are linked to one another. Quine and Ullian, two philosophers, use the metaphor of a web to describe the structure of an individual's belief system.[1] Beliefs are interwoven. They draw strength and support from one another. When we try to change pessimism into optimism, we have to remember that someone's beliefs about the future are tied to other beliefs that must be confronted as well.[2]

Psychologists have done a great deal of research trying to understand the principles that describe the particular weave of someone's web. One that emerges time and again is consistency. Indeed, some theorists even go so far as to propose that when a person perceives any sort of inconsistency among her beliefs, she experiences actual discomfort and is thereby motivated to attain consistency.[3] She does this by changing aspects of what she thinks.

Consistency is one of the basic organizational principles. And so when we plan how to change the way a person thinks, we have to be aware that we will be pushing against it. One of the perverse things about consistency is that sometimes it is preferred to good feelings. A person may sacrifice the benefits of optimism simply because it is incongruent with her other beliefs. Underlying Groucho Marx's quip that he would not belong to a club that would have him as a member is a standard operating principle among people who have low self-esteem. In some studies, there is even evidence that people with a poor opinion of themselves will go out of their way to receive feedback consistent with this low opinion: they literally search for slaps in the face.[4] Because pessimists are particularly apt to have a low opinion of their own worth and abilities, they will probably resist evidence that things are better than they take them to be. As we pointed out in Chapter 1, for many optimism has connotations of childishness and naivete. For these people, suggestions to look at the brighter side of things are apt to fall on deaf ears. If they change isolated beliefs, the change will probably be temporary because their other beliefs will lead them to "reweave" the web.

It is fortunate that beliefs can be changed indirectly—not by attacking them per se but by getting at related beliefs that in turn will affect them. Milton Rokeach is a psychologist who pioneered some intriguing ways of changing people's prejudiced racial attitudes.[5] Rather than taking on these attitudes directly, he instead encouraged prejudiced people to examine their more general values concerning freedom and equality. As these were articulated and their interdependence was appreciated, people came to see that they could not hold the value of freedom without also endorsing the value of equality. They changed their attitudes to be congruent with the values that they now recognized as their own.

An interesting fact about psychotherapy is that despite the difficulty of helping people solve particular problems, when progress is made, it is often on several fronts simultaneously, including specific ones never directly attacked in therapy sessions. Focusing on problems at home, for example, may help solve problems at work, or vice versa. This follows from our argument that beliefs are woven together. To the degree that individuals change one habitual belief, then others necessarily follow.

The other people in one's life—friends and family members—can be either disastrous or helpful, precisely because *they* have a need to maintain a consistent view of things as well. We have already discussed the contagion of pessimism. If two friends hold pessimistic views, then they are apt to stay pessimistic. If one cheers up, the other's negative view of the world is threatened. He may well act to bring his friend abruptly down to earth. Conversely, if two friends are both optimistic, their respective needs for consistency will lead them to lift one another out of occasional bad moods and negative views.

Cognitive-Behavioral Therapy

Bearing in mind these general ideas about changing beliefs, let us turn to the question of how people can change their firmly entrenched beliefs. Recent years have brought breakthroughs in the psychological treatment of emotional and behavioral difficulties. In contrast to psychoanalytic therapy, which tries to solve people's problems by exposing hidden conflicts, these new therapeutic approaches take a more pragmatic and direct approach to helping people: if someone is afraid of air travel, for example, then *that* is the problem that needs to be attacked in therapy, not whatever may lie deep beneath the surface.

These new approaches came out of either cognitive psychology or behavior modification, but they have now converged. It makes sense to describe them collectively as cognitive-behavioral therapy. They provide helpful hints for how a person might become more optimistic in his thinking and more efficacious in his actions.

Behavior modification   Behavior modification has a simple premise: people learn to behave in an "abnormal" fashion. Whatever problems they have stem from their history of rewards and punishments. Given different rewards and punishments, they learn to behave differently. And thus behavior modification provides a set of techniques for helping a client rid himself of undesired habits and replace them with desired ones. These techniques are most often used to change "behavioral" habits, but they are also useful in attacking pessimism insofar as our beliefs are entwined with our behaviors.

Behavior therapists seek to change a particular behavior of a person by manipulating its consequences. Bad habits can be eliminated by arranging matters so that the relevant behaviors are punished (i.e., followed by undesirable consequences); good habits can be strengthened by seeing to it that they are reinforced (i.e., followed by desirable consequences). This approach intervenes in a person's environment. The therapist changes the rules of the game—the prevailing pattern of punishments and rewards—thereby modifying her client's behavior.

Aversion therapy is a good example of behavior modification. In this approach, an aversive stimulus is associated with some undesirable behavior, in the hope that the client will learn to link the behavior with its new consequences and thereby refrain from performing it. For example, alcohol might be mixed with a drug that makes him feel nauseous. Someone with a deviant sexual impulse—like one that involves children—might have his inappropriate sexual responses followed by electric shock.

Or, in the case of a child who never shares with other children, never follows her parent's suggestions, never does her homework, and never walks the dog, a behavior therapist would look not to the child for an explanation of these actions but rather to her environment. Perhaps her parents inadvertently reward precisely those behaviors that so upset them by paying attention to her when she behaves badly. When she happens to behave well, her parents ignore her or—even worse—heap unpleasant demands upon her.

Training the parents is one possible solution: teaching *them* how to respond to their child. They should reward her for behaviors they wish to increase and not reward her for behaviors they wish to decrease. Now, all of this may seem perfectly obvious. Surely most parents know that praise is more effective than punishment. But watching parents respond to their children in any crowded store, one realizes the discrepancy between theory and practice. At any rate, parent training and similar procedures have proven highly effective in changing children's behavior.[6]

Behavior modifiers also use techniques based on observational learning,[7] described in Chapter 3. A client's problems can be solved by having him watch models, either on film or in person, successfully cope with whatever overwhelms him. Fears and phobias can be eliminated this way. For example, modeling has been used to reduce people's fears about entering a hospital for surgery. If a patient sees a film of another patient who went through a similar surgical procedure without fear, he experiences less apprehension himself.[8]

There is quite a mythology surrounding behavior modification, so let us dispel a few of the false ideas that some hold. It is *not* an all-powerful strategy for making anyone do anything the behavior therapist wants. It has its share of failures, particularly as a treatment for substance abuse.[9] Further, behavior therapy is *not* dehumanizing. Perhaps brief descriptions of its procedures, like the ones presented here, are responsible for this misconception. Out of context, the techniques seem cold and mechanical. But behavior therapists are *not* technicians. They are first and foremost therapists, which means they deploy their strategies within a therapeutic relationship.

The biggest limitation of traditional behavior modification is that it ignores the client's mental life. As we have been emphasizing throughout this book, thoughts and beliefs are important determinants of feelings and actions, and so behavior modification is necessarily incomplete until the mutual influence between thought and behavior is acknowledged. We are hardly the first to point this out, and indeed, behavior therapists are now beginning to explicitly address cognitive factors in their rationale and procedures. Other therapeutic approaches have focused more explicitly on people's thoughts as determinants of their behavior. Let us consider two of the best-known therapies that are cognitive in nature.

Rational-emotive therapy   Rational-emotive therapy was developed by psychologist Albert Ellis.[10] Ellis believes that people make trouble for themselves by how they think about things. They tend to entertain irrational beliefs that necessarily make them anxious or depressed or otherwise troubled. Consider these beliefs:

- I *must* do well at everything I try.
- I *must* be loved and respected by everyone I know.
- I *must* be completely happy all the time.
- I *must* get my way with other people.

Ellis calls this tendency "musturbation" and argues that someone who holds such rigid beliefs has a poor road map for navigating the world.

When faced with a client who makes such statements, the rational-emotive therapist actively disputes them. Therapy is therefore quite directive. On the face of it, the therapist is argumentative, but "arguments" occur in the context of an accepting relationship. He disputes her beliefs, not the client herself.

> CLIENT: I feel discouraged about life these days.
> THERAPIST: It sounds like you think no one should be discouraged.
> CLIENT: Well, being discouraged is a drag. I can't stand it.
> THERAPIST: I'd agree that discouragement is no fun, but don't confuse your wants with your needs.
> Why do you say you can't stand discouragement? You've survived pretty well so far.
> CLIENT: But when I wake up in the morning, the only thing I look forward to during the whole day is going to sleep again that night!
> THERAPIST: Do you really mean that?

Research shows that rational-emotive therapy helps people with pervasive anxiety disorders, although there is disagreement over the effectiveness of argument per se.[11] We believe that this technique works because the therapist cares about his clients—not because he disputes their beliefs.

Cognitive therapy   A final therapy, also thoroughly cognitive, is the one developed by psychiatrist Aaron Beck,[12] appropriately called cognitive therapy. We discussed Beck's theory of depression in Chapter 5, and his therapy stems from its central premise that particular ways of thinking may produce difficulties for someone. Like other cognitive approaches, Beck's therefore tries to change a person's particular thoughts, on the assumption that modifying thoughts will reduce depression and anxiety. He describes cognitive therapy as "collaborative empiricism" to emphasize that the therapist and client work together (collaborate) to check the client's beliefs against the facts of the matter (empiricism).

The first step in cognitive therapy is to identify the client's automatic thoughts, the habitual putdowns that flash through her mind in the course of a typical day. The therapist asks his client to pay attention to these thoughts, and not just to the emotional damage they cause. She is encouraged to write them down, along with the feelings they produce. Then she is asked to challenge each automatic thought by asking what evidence she has for believing it:

> I got depressed at work when the boss walked by me without saying hello. My thoughts were that I did a lousy job on my last project, that he was mad at me, and that I was probably going to be fired.
>
> But when I think further about that incident, I guess I can see that my boss was probably preoccupied. His son has been ill. Plus I've done projects like that before, with good results. And I got a raise just two months ago.

The process of cognitive therapy is more difficult than our example conveys. Automatic thoughts can be elusive, and they are so common that a client does not even notice them. And even when she does, she finds out that automatic thoughts are not simply errors like mistaken telephone numbers that can be readily corrected once she attends to them. Rather, these thoughts are deeply embedded. Clients challenge them only with great reluctance. Recognizing the difficulty of changing such beliefs, cognitive therapists often devise experiments to help their clients challenge what they believe.

"You think you're a social loser? Maybe yes, maybe no. Why don't you find out by asking ten different people to have a cup of coffee with you? Keep track of how many people say yes. And tell me before you start how many people would have to accept your invitation for you *not* to be a loser." Needless to say, the therapist must use some common sense in these assignments and not send an accountant off to party with the Hell's Angels. But maladaptive beliefs can be effectively challenged if the experiences are appropriately chosen.

Usually, cognitive therapy involves weekly sessions over several months. Research shows that the procedure effectively alleviates depression as well as various anxiety disorders.[13] It also holds promise for people who suffer from chronic pain, obesity, marital strife, and eating disorders. Shortly, we will describe a study that shows how cognitive therapy can turn pessimists into optimists.

Commonalities   What do these therapies tell us about the way to go about changing one's habits and beliefs? First, there is a common emphasis on reality. Beliefs must be tested. The world in which one lives—and here we mean in particular the social world—must be hospitable to what one is trying to do. If it is to think more optimistically, a person cannot do this and maintain close relations with pessimists.

Second, there is a common emphasis on activity; these therapies all stress that change does not occur in a passive person. Sometimes the person must go out and learn new skills.

- So, you're not socially adept? We'll figure out how you can do better.
- What? You don't know how to plan ahead for a better future? Well, let's figure out how to do that as well.

Many times, people have to express and justify the beliefs that they have. And sometimes the best way to do that is to see whether they prove useful as they navigate the real world.

Third, there is a common emphasis on the therapeutic relationship. Another person—the therapist—is helpful in devising the process of belief change and guiding the person through it. Is a therapist needed to become more optimistic? We think not, but if people want to challenge or change a belief, they must do so in a social context. A therapist is specifically trained to create the circumstances for this change, and a person working alone will be hard pressed to be as successful. We will later sketch strategies someone can use without a therapist to become more optimistic, but they do entail other people as allies.

Fourth, there is a common emphasis on the avoidance of black-white dichotomies. If someone adopts rigidly optimistic beliefs and expects *only* good things, his belief system will be too brittle. During therapy, one should expect change to be gradual. There will be setbacks and occasions when the world is indeed dark and gloomy. That is the nature of change as well as life itself: three steps forward, two backward, and list to the side. Forward progress should be the trend, however.

Studies of psychotherapy suggest that while as many as one out of five Americans will seek out therapy at some point, of this group, as many as 80% will stop before therapy is complete. The primary culprit appears to be dashed expectations. The general public is correctly told that therapy works, but perhaps they should additionally be told what "working" means. Successful therapy means improvement in some problem area, but it does not mean miraculous overnight transformations. People may well expect them, become disappointed, and drop out of therapy.

Suppose someone is depressed and gloomy seven days out of seven. Suppose therapy is effective to the extent that he begins to feel poorly only four days out of seven. Some might brand this outcome as disappointing and the therapy a failure. But we prefer to see it as an improvement.

Fifth, there is agreement that goals in therapy should be modest and immediate. If they are too vast or too distant, the person will feel overwhelmed. Consider attempts at losing weight. If a person wants to lose fifty pounds, it may seem impossible because fifty pounds is an imposing amount. But if she only wants to lose two pounds the first week, she can handle it. Then she sets a new goal. The principle for changing one's beliefs from pessimistic to optimistic is the same. Conceive the task as a series of small steps. No one gains fifty pounds, and no one becomes a pessimist, overnight. So why should anyone approach weight loss or belief change as if it could take place quickly?

Sixth, there is a common emphasis on specificity. The underlying principle is that to change particular problems, the individual must set particular goals and use particular techniques. Therapy is not a situation in which people sit and talk vaguely about the meaning of life, but rather one in which they address concrete thoughts and actions in concrete situations.

Seventh, there is a common belief that the person must be treated as an integrated whole. His thoughts relate to one another. His thoughts relate to his actions and vice versa. And his thoughts and beliefs are tied to events in his world.

Eighth, there is a common concern that the client need not be kept in the dark about the processes of change. Clients can and should be enlisted as active assistants in the process. A previous generation of therapists may have believed in the importance of therapeutic distance, but contemporary cognitive-behavioral therapists do *not* mystify the business of how to change beliefs. They encourage their clients to read books about therapy, to ask questions, and to make suggestions about how to proceed.

Finally, there is a common emphasis on hope: the positive expectation that makes any sort of psychotherapy possible. There is a tension here. People seek out therapy when they are demoralized in the face of some problem. But they also have to believe that they can be helped. This puts a considerable burden on the therapist, to accept the concern of the client while at the same time holding out the promise of improvement. Indeed, many suggest that the attitude of a therapist is much more important than the specific techniques that he or she uses. We suggest that optimism is a critical aspect of the preferred therapeutic attitude.

Specific Investigations

We have been discussing belief change in general and how therapy can bring it about. But what do we know about the actual circumstances in which people begin to think more (or less) optimistically? We will now turn to some studies that have documented changes in people's explanatory style, from optimistic to pessimistic and from pessimistic to optimistic. First, two case studies show how a series of bad events chip away at one's optimism.

The Baltimore Orioles and Freud   The 1988 baseball season was a disaster for the Baltimore Orioles team. The season started with a record-setting 21 straight losses by the team. It seemed that no matter what the players or coaching staff did, the team lost. We saw this as an opportunity to study the effects of protracted bad events on explanatory style—in this case the "collective" style of the entire team.

We obtained the hometown paper of the Orioles and read each story about the Orioles during this streak.[14] We used the CAVE technique described in Chapter 1 to identify and rate each causal explanation made by an Orioles player about a lost game. See Table 7–1 for some examples. Raters who did not know which game each quote applied to then rated each causal explanation as optimistic or pessimistic. As we suspected, the longer the streak went on, the more pessimistic the players became.[15]

In another case study of how a series of bad events can take a toll on someone's optimism we studied the way that psychoanalyst Sigmund Freud explained events.[16] We drew on his voluminous published correspondence, and read letters by Freud that spanned decades. When we encountered bad events and explanations for them, we coded them for optimism versus pessimism with the CAVE technique.

Freud's later years were not happy ones. Although he received increasing fame and acclaim, he was also faced with a series of per-

TABLE 7–1. *Causal Explanations by the Baltimore Orioles*

Earlier in losing streak

The wind was blowing in . . . and we just picked a bad night to hit some balls good.

I had a good bead on it when it was hit . . . I looked up to catch it, and [because] the sun was on my right side, I just lost it.

Sometimes you have games like that . . . The positive thing is we're going to show up [tomorrow], and the score will be 0–0.

We'll bounce back . . . every team has games like this.

Another tough game . . . [because] we're asking our pitchers to throw a shutout every night.

We're going to turn it around sometime, but it's not as quickly as anyone thought.

It's [the umpires'] game . . . they control it. They call them when they want to.

It's a test . . . it's a real test.

There's tremendous pressure. It's not a monkey on our backs anymore. It's Godzilla.

because we don't have a leadoff hitter.

They know they played poorly . . . I don't have to call a meeting to tell them that.

We've got all the excuses, the weather, not getting the breaks, but it's still just losing.

Later in losing streak

sonal tragedies. He suffered from cancer of the mouth and underwent 27 different operations. He lost two sons in World War One. The rise of Nazism was an incredible horror. Many of Freud's close relatives were sent to concentration camps where they perished. His books were seized and burned by the Nazis. He had to flee his native Vienna at the very end of his life and seek refuge in England.

Biographers of Freud are unanimous in concluding that he was not a happy person. Actual life events obviously affect how one feels (Chapter 3), and Freud's moods darkened as the bad experiences started to accumulate. His psychoanalytic theory did not suggest an optimistic perspective on the human condition to begin with, but we were interested in whether his pessimism showed up on a day-to-day basis in his correspondence, and if it increased in response to the disasters just mentioned.

Our analyses of his causal explanations with the CAVE technique show that this is exactly what happened. Freud became ever more pessimistic as he became older. His representative causal explanations over the last few years of his life indicate a clear trend toward pessimism (see Table 7–2).

An interesting aspect of Freud's attributions was that as he became older, he increasingly used his age to explain why bad events occurred. Children also use age to explain things, but of course children will someday be older. Whatever the reality basis of so-called age attributions by the elderly, they are not useful because they are fatal-

TABLE 7–2. *Causal Explanations by Sigmund Freud*

Earlier in his career

Feeling miserable . . . [because] drinking sugar water.

Can't provide useful information on Nietzsche . . . [because] friend overestimates my knowledge of Nietzsche.

Didn't publish book . . . [because] my opinion about the weakness of my historical construction was confirmed.

I can't produce anything new . . . [because] this time of life [old age].

I'm unlikely to see this friend again . . . [because] I'm approaching life's inevitable end.

No longer want to write . . . [because] unproductiveness of old age.

Later in his career

istic. They rationalize passivity. In terms of our perspective, causal explanations of this sort are among the most pessimistic that can be entertained because old age cannot—by definition—be reversed.

Along these lines, Margie Lachman of Brandeis University has made a systematic study of optimistic and pessimistic explanatory styles among the elderly.[17] Her results converge with our analysis here. When people who are elderly explain bad events in terms of their age, they behave more helplessly. They also report more health problems.[18]

A different approach to aging and the limitations that it may impose is offered by the behaviorist B. F. Skinner. In an intriguing account, he described some of the adjustments he made to his old age. He started with the provocative point that not only do people age, but so too do their environments. Some of the problems of old age can thus be combated by changing the environment. If one is forgetful, one can leave reminders:

> Ten minutes before you leave your house for the day you hear a weather report: It will probably rain before you return. It occurs to you to take an umbrella . . . [but] ten minutes later you leave without the umbrella. You can solve that kind of problem by executing as much of the behavior as possible when it occurs to you. Hang the umbrella on the doorknob, or put it through the handle of your briefcase, or in some other way start the process of taking it with you.[19]

Needless to say, not only the aged can benefit from this strategy of remembering.

As a behaviorist, Skinner has no use for mentalistic notions like optimism or pessimism, but it is nonetheless possible to describe his approach in this example as the epitome of optimism. It is future oriented, reality based, and manifest in active behavior. He confronted the problem of forgetfulness by devising a solution to it.

Explanatory style and therapy We know that cognitive-behavioral therapy is an effective way to change someone's explanatory style from pessimistic to optimistic. In a study by Martin Seligman and others at the University of Pennsylvania, 39 depressed patients undergoing therapy at the Center for Cognitive Therapy—run by Aaron Beck—were followed over the course of therapy and one year afterward.[20]

On the average, these 39 patients were seen once a week over a six month period, which resulted in about 22 sessions per patient. A comparison group of 10 "normal" (nonpatient) individuals was recruited through the media and matched to patients in terms of sex, age, and education. The purpose of this comparison group was to rule out any explanations in terms merely of the passage of time.

Explanatory style was measured with the ASQ at three points in time—at the beginning of therapy, at the end of therapy (i.e., after six months of successful treatment), and then one year following termination. This study is continuing, so we will be able to learn about the even longer-term consequences of therapy for optimism and pessimism. But what Seligman and his colleagues have discovered to date is already highly encouraging.

As we would expect, the patients started therapy with a pessimistic explanatory style—in comparison to the nonpatient comparison group. Their explanatory style improved from pessimistic to optimistic in the course of therapy. Indeed, the more optimistic they became, the greater was the extent to which their depression lifted. The gains in optimism, on the whole, were maintained over the one year follow-up period. There was some erosion—toward pessimism and depression—among some patients one year after the end of therapy, and these were most likely to be patients who were somewhat pessimistic at the time that their therapy originally ended. In other words, pessimism breeds pessimism, just as optimism produces further optimism.

There is an obvious chicken-egg problem here, because depression and pessimism moved in lockstep during and after therapy. In a way, this is not surprising, granted the link between the two (as discussed in Chapter 5). But as a result, we do not know the exact process by which cognitive therapy transforms pessimism into optimism. For instance, it may directly affect someone's pessimistic beliefs for the better. Or cognitive therapy may first improve a patient's mood, which in turn changes her pessimistic attitude.

But in a way, the details do not matter, if the point is that people can become more optimistic as a function of the sorts of experiences they encounter during therapy. Elsewhere, we have presented considerable evidence for the stability of optimism or pessimism, so this is an important demonstration.

Two questions still remain about changing beliefs from pessimistic to optimistic via therapy. The first stems from the fact that the Seligman study investigated pessimistic depressives. Does cognitive therapy similarly work to change the beliefs of pessimistic *non-*

depressives? We simply do not know at the present time, although we can argue both pro and con.

On the one hand, it might be easier to change the pessimism of depressives simply because their depression tends to lift in the course of therapy, and this is a tremendous boost. The successful treatment of depression provides many clues to a person that he is capable. He feels better—not just in terms of his mood but his body as well; he is more energetic and alert; and he rediscovers appetites long dormant. All of these changes should bolster his optimism. Clients may well regard a successful bout with depression as a major mastery experience, one that underscores their ability to have an impact on matters in general.

On the other hand, depressives tend to think in exactly the sorts of ways that make optimism difficult to encourage via therapeutic techniques.[21] Depressives view the world in black-white terms. They selectively attend to evidence that supports their negative view of themselves. They have the bleakest expectations for the future. And they use "illogical" justifications for their pessimistic beliefs.

To illustrate: with Michelle Cook, we interviewed severely depressed individuals.[22] We gave them a version of the Attributional Style Questionnaire in interview form—asking them to describe bad events and then to explain why they had happened. But then we asked them what their evidence was for believing that the cause they cited—which was invariably a pessimistic one—was the one that was operative. When compared to a group of nondepressed individuals, the depressives were strikingly irrational.

Although we were not in a position to evaluate the "truth" of the causes they cited, we could still see if they at least appeared in principle to be adequate explanations. A causal explanation should specify some cause that precedes the event in question and presumably brings about that event. In the absence of the cause, the event would not take place. Nondepressed individuals usually cited explanations of this sort. Depressed individuals almost never did.

Instead, they might restate the event as "evidence" for the cause: "My boyfriend dropped me [bad event] because I'm not a good person [cause], and I know I'm not a good person because he dropped me [evidence?]." Or they pulled a *non sequitur* out of thin air: "I flunked the course [bad event] because the teacher didn't like women [cause]; he once told a woman in class to be quiet [evidence?]." Or sometimes they simply drew a blank. These moments were poignant. Our research subjects would stare at us when we asked *why* they believed that something they said was a cause, and they would slowly shake their heads. "I don't have the slightest idea why I believe that. But that's what I believe."

The point is that depressed pessimists may be difficult to treat because their characteristic way of thinking works precisely in a way to maintain their pessimism. Nondepressed pessimists may be easier to help using the techniques of cognitive-behavioral therapy because they have more capabilities at their disposal.

Further research is needed. Most importantly, we need to know if cognitive-behavioral techniques are effective in changing pessimists into optimists when they are not depressed to begin with. Our hunch—an optimistic one, to be sure—is that these techniques will work at least as well with the nondepressed and quite likely they will work better. We do know from the study of educational challenge described in Chapter 4 that "normal" individuals can become more optimistic in their ways of thinking if they are given encouragement and mastery experiences.

The second question that remains is what the long-range effects on physical health might be of changing one's way of thinking from pessimistic to optimistic. We know that optimism is more closely linked with better health than is pessimism. And we also know that people can change their way of thinking from pessimistic to optimistic. What we do not know is whether we can put these two facts together and conclude that born-again optimism confers the same benefits on physical well-being as does optimism present all along.[23]

Even if the answer is yes, we should not expect immediate health benefits from a change to optimism. A friend who works in a hospital with coronary patients likes to point out that she has never talked to a patient on her ward who smokes. They all proudly claim to be ex-smokers. She has learned to ask them *when* they gave up the practice, and they often tell her, with a straight face, that the last cigarette they had was during the initial stages of their heart attack.

Becoming an optimist at a later point in life is similarly unlikely to bring immediate benefits. It takes time for one's optimism to have an effect on one's physiology, on one's habitual mood, on one's perseverance in the face of adversity, and on one's social relationships.

Seligman's investigation of patients whose explanatory style became more optimistic as a result of cognitive therapy will provide us with important information as they are followed through time. Will their health start to improve? If so, when will this improvement start to show itself? Will certain symptoms and illnesses be more or less sensitive to an increase in optimism? Again, evidence like this can be used to specify more exactly the sorts of pathways that link optimism and physical well-being.

Specific Things to Do

For several years, we have been giving interviews to writers of popular magazines about the relationship between optimism and health. They listen politely to the details of the actual studies and to our careful qualifications about what we can and cannot conclude from them. But we imagine they really care little about the methodological and theoretical subtleties. After they have heard us out, all of them cut to the same bottom line: "What can someone do in order to be more optimistic?" After many interviews,[24] we have generated a set of reasonable do's and don't's.

As we have seen earlier in this chapter, however, belief change is not a simple enterprise. Beliefs—optimistic or pessimistic—cohere with the other ideas that one entertains, and undesirable beliefs cannot be excised neatly and cleanly, and simply replaced with desirable ones. At different points in life we are more versus less open to challenging our belief systems, and we cannot push a process that is not ready to take place. And change takes place slowly, only with effort.

What should someone do who wants to change?

1. *Choose an area of life in which to become more optimistic:* perhaps work or family or friends or the future or health. The list is endless, but one has to make a choice and be specific. It is necessary to stand someplace in order to paint the floor. Not everything can be changed at once. A good choice to make is an area that is important enough to demand attention and concern but not so critical that the thought of change frightens one into inaction.

2. *Become mindful of his thoughts with respect to this area of life.* First, he must listen to himself. What are the sorts of pessimistic things he says in the course of the day? What broader assumptions does his pessimism rest upon? (This is of course the procedure involved in Beck's identification of automatic thoughts.) He should write these down as he says them. He will probably be amazed at how frequently pessimistic they are. It may turn out that pessimism is attached to particular settings and circumstances—as when a deadline looms at work. Such information is valuable in mounting the campaign for change.

3. *Consider the reality of the beliefs he espouses.* What evidence does he have for believing pessimistic things about this area of his life? If he finds that his evidence is inadequate, his beliefs may become more optimistic. If he finds that reality is indeed grim, he must take steps to reprogram the world so that optimistic beliefs are plausible; this means avoiding negative people and situations. He may have to accept that certain events are beyond his control. If he has interviewed for a new job and is waiting to hear the result, then the die is cast. Fretting about the past, present, or future will have no bearing on the result of the already completed interview.

4. *Set modest and immediate goals with respect to changes in his optimism.* He should resolve, for instance, to cut self-deprecating statements at work in two by the end of next week. He should keep track of his progress in a way that allows him to *see* change. Pessimists need to be convinced that things are improving, so they should buy pencils and paper and make charts.

5. *Give himself rewards when his modest goals are met.* Here he needs to identify things he really likes to do—perhaps going out to dinner, or reading a novel straight through, or staying up late to watch a talk show. He should be good to himself, however he defines that, when he has earned it.

6. *Seek out optimistic people.* Pessimism cannot be eradicated from the world, but someone seeking to change can still exert some influence on what and whom he exposes himself to. If someone who cannot be avoided insists on being negative despite all attempts to urge or suggest more positive views, we recommend a tactic sketched by Eric Berne in his book *Games People Play.*[25]

The game Berne calls "Why Don't You, Yes But," is one of the favorite activities of pessimists. They bring up a problem to someone, apparently asking for possible solutions. To every sincere suggestion that is offered ("Why don't you . . . "), they respond with a putdown ("Yes but . . . "), subverting the suggestion and rationalizing their further pessimism and inactivity. Eventually, the would-be helper joins them in gloom; he has proven himself as ineffective at solving their problems as they are.

The human inclination is to help someone who has a problem, but if she resists help, then this becomes a game that can never be won. The pessimist is the judge and jury for any suggestion, and she has already decided the case. To "win" this game with a pessimist,

Berne suggests listening carefully and then saying, "That's quite a problem! What are *you* going to do about it?"

7. *Play at being optimistic.* We mean this in two senses. The person seeking to change should create a role for himself as an optimistic person, and then act it out.[26] He may find it easier to play such a role by going out among people who do not know him, to be unencumbered by expectations. Sometimes a new role can be boosted in the way that real actors enhance their roles—by method acting techniques. Someone might remember past moments of optimism and try to recreate those thoughts and feelings. Or he might change his style of clothing or how he combs his hair. If he gives his system a jolt, perhaps his web of belief will loosen up enough for him to weave a yellow ribbon through it.

The person trying to change the way he thinks should have fun in the process. He should literally play at it. Becoming optimistic is a serious effort, to be sure, but not a deadly serious one. The person seeking to change should adopt an attitude of adventure. Or he should make fun of himself, either for being an aspiring optimist or for being pessimistic in the first place.

8. *Remember that optimism is healthy inasmuch as it catalyzes actions.* The person seeking to change should behave in accordance with his growing optimism, devising solutions to problems, being resourceful, helping other people, cultivating hobbies. Productive activity will generate further optimism.

We often talk to our students about their career choices. Many are confused because they want work that interests them, but they are not sure what this might be. We undertake a gentle form of Socratic sarcasm:

> What do you really like to eat?
> Okay, you really like chocolate cake.
> Can you imagine ever not liking chocolate cake in the future?
> Wouldn't it be nice if you had a career as rewarding as chocolate cake?
> How did you know that you would like chocolate cake?
> Did you sit around and puzzle it out before you had any?
> You say you tried it first?
> You probably tried other things, too, like carrot cake.
> But you found out that you liked chocolate cake better.
> Then why don't you choose a career the same way?

Experimenting is important. Interests are not generated in an internal dialogue while sitting alone at home. Thus too, one does not just talk oneself into optimism; one must go out and act optimistically and let "beliefs" catch up to actions.

9. *Refrain from doing all of this in a social vacuum.* Someone seeking to change should find a friend with whom he can plot a strategy to become more optimistic. Needless to say, it should be a good friend. They should talk all of this over, devising strategies for change and procedures for evaluating success. He should ask his friend to reward his triumphs, and kick him when he falls short. He needs encouragement but not commiseration. He should avoid anyone who will tell him how terrible things are. This is not the sort of social support that encourages optimism.

10. *Appreciate that becoming optimistic entails a lifestyle change.* Optimism is not something that a person can work on for a few days and master. An obvious parallel is with bad physical habits. It is rather easy to start to change such habits. In the short run most people can give up smoking or drinking, or lose some weight. But in the short run the person is mindful, progress is novel, and incentives are high. In the short run becoming an optimist is also easy, as those who played Pollyanna's glad game demonstrated. The difficulty lies in making the change permanent.

Bizarre diets are not a good idea. People cannot stay on them indefinitely. It is the *maintenance* that is the real challenge. Likewise, optimism must be integrated into one's everyday thinking so that the change is permanent. Backsliding—although normal in the process of change—may be particularly insidious if the person uses it as "proof" for his pessimism. "I knew it wouldn't work." Also, some of the extreme efforts to change beliefs, as found in encounter groups or cults, might well be effective in the short run, but such mechanisms for change are too unusual to keep in place for very long. Hence, erosion is inevitable.

11. *Approach this task in a flexible way.* There will be inevitable setbacks. Sometimes it will be impossible to be optimistic. Sometimes bad things will happen, and the person seeking to change will feel foolish for expecting the best. Sometimes other people will tease him. Such problems can be handled if they have been anticipated. A person should try to make a small change if a big one is impossible. He should recast disappointments as challenges. Or he should find another area of life to savor.

Becoming on Optimist *and* Becoming Healthy

Again, we do not advocate an all-out effort to become an immediate across-the-board optimist. Changes in one domain of life will have benefits elsewhere, but thoughts have to be attacked one at a time. Might one choose health as a focus? By all means. "Healthful living" means various things, but usually it is directed at reducing one of the established risk factors for poor health, like stress or dietary fat or alcohol consumption.

So, one may become healthier first by becoming more optimistic, then by letting optimism make one more attractive to others, then by enjoying relationships with these people, and finally by reaping the benefits of these relationships in terms of the physical well-being they produce. But one need not start this chain of events by becoming more optimistic. One can just as well start by becoming more attractive. Indeed, this should lead not only more directly to good health but can additionally feed back and boost optimism which will then boost health.

The promise of a long life may not be incentive enough for doing something in the here and now. Long-term "health" grimly pursued may be a questionable goal because it is too distant.[27] A person needs incentives along the way.[28]

The voluminous health promotion literature demands sophisticated psychological theory to explain why an individual's attempts to reduce risk factors meet with success or failure.[29] Oversimplified views of human nature have often prevailed. People are seen in one of two opposite yet equally unrealistic ways, either as objects who can be passively pushed around by information contained in public service announcements or as agents infinitely responsive to any and all exhortations to be healthy.

The facts are complex, and this probably explains why all health promotion efforts—diets, campaigns to reduce cholesterol, stress management programs, and the like—have at best mixed success. They reach some people but not others.[30] They tend to leave the person out of the formula, and in particular they neglect the person's characteristic optimism and pessimism with respect to the target of the healthy practice being pushed. A pessimist is not going to be moved by information or exhortation. "Why bother?" Health promoters should remember that it is people who adopt the practices that are good or bad for health, that people have characteristic beliefs, and that these beliefs determine which of their behaviors can be changed and how this can be done.

CHAPTER

8

Taking Stock

Be not afraid of life. Believe that
life is worth living, and your belief
will help create the fact.
— *William James*

W e have made the following general points:

- Optimism should not be regarded as an exercise in fantasy, but as a reality-based belief system that leads us to be active and effective in our lives, working toward good outcomes while avoiding bad ones.
- One way to assess people's characteristic levels of optimism is to ascertain their explanatory style: how they habitually explain bad events.
- Various studies show that an optimistic explanatory style is associated with good health; a pessimistic explanatory style with poor health.
- Other studies support these findings, showing generally that positive thoughts are associated with physical well-being.
- Optimism originates in childhood. Its association with good health appears to be mediated via several routes—physiological, emotional, behavioral, and interpersonal—that intersect one another.
- People can become more optimistic as adults and, we would predict, thereby reap some of the benefits that accompany optimism, including good health.

Along the way, we have noted unanswered questions as well as problems and gaps in the evidence.

In a very literal sense, this book is a progress report on a research program that is still unfinished. The future will take researchers both inward, to learn more about how psychological factors influence the nervous system, endocrine system, and immune system and eventually determine physical well-being, as well as outward—to locate optimism and health in their societal context.

Looking Back

Our own studies continue a line of investigations of how mind and body influence each other that goes back many hundreds of years. A review of these investigations underscores how far we have come in understanding possible psychological influences on health. Some of the turning points in the history of thinking about the relationship between mind and body are described here.

Ancient times   A reasonable place to start *any* Western intellectual history is with the work of Aristotle. His famous description *mens sana in corpore sano* ("a healthy mind in a healthy body") suggests that some 2500 years ago the idea was explicit that mental and physical well-being are closely entwined.

The influence ran both ways, from mind to body and from body to mind. For centuries, literature and art in Western Europe frequently equated physical prowess and beauty with a strong and virtuous character. These stereotypes persist to this day, as evidenced on movie screens and in research reports of social psychologists who study the effects of good looks on the impressions we form of others.

The early physicians—Hippocrates (460–377 B.C.), Galen (129–199), and others—never doubted that minds and bodies exerted a mutual influence. Part of medical practice at its very inception involved ministering to the patient's entire being, addressing what we now call psychological factors as well as treating specific illnesses and injuries. The individuality of a patient was never overlooked.

The 1600s   Rene Descartes (1596–1650) was a French intellectual variously honored as the founder of physiological psychology, the creator of mathematical physics, the inventor of analytic geometry, an important contributor to optics, and a major philosopher. One of his legacies to the modern world was his strong stance concerning the dualism of the mind and body.[1]

As a young man living in Paris, Descartes would wander through the parks where mechanized statues were the rage. As pedestrians stepped on a plate on the walkway, it would trigger a hydraulic device that forced water through underground pipes into the limbs of the nearby statues, causing them to move and dance. If mechanized beings worked this way, he thought, then why not human beings? Descartes knew that the brain contained hollow spaces filled with fluid, that tubes (that is, nerves) led from the brain to all the other parts of the body, and that muscles swelled as they were used. He therefore proposed that our bodies moved when the brain sent fluid to the appropriate muscles.

Descartes' theory of movement correctly discerned the role of the nervous system in making movement possible as well as the controlling and coordinating functions of the brain. He was wrong about the mechanism, and his hydraulic ideas have since been supplanted by theories stressing electrical and chemical processes.

Wrong in details, but right in overall thrust, his theory was phrased in the language of modern science, pointing to causes and effects. But his work led him into conflict with prevailing opinion. In proposing that people obeyed the same deterministic laws as the rest of the universe, Descartes in effect was ignoring the doctrine of free will, the notion that people's actions were freely chosen and hence could not reflect causes—hydraulic, electrical, or chemical. To ignore free will was to invite trouble with the Church.

Aware of the danger, Descartes was careful in how he phrased his theory. Our bodies are subject to physical laws, he argued, and hence bodily functions can be thought of as having causes. But our souls are free and do not fall under a deterministic umbrella. Thus, bodies and souls were split apart more for political reasons than scientific ones. Because of the forcefulness of his distinction, and because other intellectuals took it seriously, wholly different vocabularies and scientific traditions (like medicine on the one hand and philosophy and then psychology on the other) were developed to study these two aspects of people. In the twentieth century, the amalgamation of these aspects in the attempt to explain how psychological states might influence health is bridging conceptual and professional chasms that have existed for centuries. Needless to say, battles ensue, such as those described in Chapter 3.

The 1700s   The eighteenth century was an intellectually vibrant one. One of its more colorful figures was Franz Anton Mesmer (1734–

1815), who might have been regarded as the founding father of modern psychiatry, were it not for the fact that he was widely seen as a charlatan and a stage artist in his own time. Mesmer was a physician, originally from Vienna, who devised a complex theory of the universe which he used to explain physical illness. He proposed that the universe—including living beings—was filled with an invisible fluid called animal magnetism. However, this fluid was not distributed evenly. Some people apparently had more than others. The former were healthy and happy, vibrant, and charismatic. The later were weak and spindly, prone to illness.

Mesmer believed that he could redistribute animal magnetism and thereby restore health to someone who was ill due to an imbalance. He devised a host of techniques, many quite flamboyant. He and his followers might form a circle, holding hands, and thereby concentrating their animal magnetism in order to relay it to one of his patients through a mere touch. Or he used a device called a baquet for accumulating animal magnetism from the atmosphere. Or he would induce a trance in an individual, make a suggestion that her symptoms would vanish, and indeed, they would!

Mesmer took his techniques from Vienna to Paris to find an appreciative audience. His cures became widely known and celebrated, so much so that a Royal Commission, composed of leading scientists (including Benjamin Franklin, then the ambassador to France, and Joseph Guillotin, the man who invented the ultimate cure for headaches), was appointed to investigate the theory of animal magnetism and the techniques that it rationalized. The Commission invalidated the theory, finding no evidence for it. However, they did not question the fact of the cures, stating instead that they were due to the imagination of the patients. Unscathed by these conclusions, Mesmer's techniques—collectively termed mesmerism—passed into general use.

It comes as no surprise that the learned men of the day debunked Mesmer's theory. He was experiencing phenomenal success. Had the number of his supporters continued to grow, traditional medical practitioners would eventually have suffered noticeable financial loss.[2]

As it turned out, mesmerism was not abandoned. These techniques became what we now call hypnotism. Why? Like Descartes, Mesmer was wrong in details, but right in overall thrust. One could argue that animal magnetism (the invisible, magical fluid) is—metaphorically—the body's natural ability to heal itself. And one could also argue that the use of an impressive device (his baquet), coupled with a physician's touch and an induced trance, could trigger healing through psychological routes. Hypnotism soon became a favored form of treatment by French psychiatrists, despite their earlier criticism of Mesmer and his cures.

1780–1850   The so-called Age of Heroic Medicine began late in the eighteenth century. The name refers to the aggressive and risky practices of orthodox medicine, as taught at the leading medical schools. If nothing else, this era shows that traditional physicians should not have been so quick to judge the practices of one of their contemporaries, Mesmer, when their own treatments bordered on the barbaric and bizarre.

Orthodox doctors at this time believed that many illnesses were caused by bad blood. Get rid of the bad blood, and one would be rid of the disease and its symptoms. How was this done? A doctor would take a sharp instrument, and cut into the patient's vein, draining away a pint of blood or more. At various intervals throughout the day and night, he repeated the procedure. Unbelievable as it may now seem in retrospect, this practice went on for years without any research to support its effectiveness.

Bleeding may have been the favorite medical practice of the day, but it certainly was not the only one:

> Intestinal purging was held in high esteem, and the drug most often used to produce it was calomel (mercurous chloride). Heroic doctors gave their patients huge doses of calomel . . . until the patient began to salivate freely, a sign that a drug was working. Toxicology tests today list salivation as an early sign of acute mercury intoxication, one of the most dangerous forms of heavy metal poisoning.
>
> In addition to purging, vomiting was induced by giving violent emetic drugs such as tartar emetic, a poisonous antimony salt. Other drugs, called diaphoretics, were used to cause profuse sweating. Blistering was carried out by rubbing or burning local irritants on the skin, including cantharides (Spanish fly). In "cupping," a heated glass cup was placed on the skin; as it cooled, a partial vacuum drew blood to the site, which was then lanced as another way of drawing off the bad fluid.[3]

By the late 1840s, the public had had enough.[4] People began a serious protest against heroic medicine in what we now call the Popular Health Movement. Because orthodox medicine could not conceive healing in terms other than bleeding and purging, the public took its chances elsewhere. Many people sought out physicians who practiced "unorthodox" medicine, like homeopathy (healing based on the administration of highly dilute forms of natural substances, like plant extracts), osteopathy (healing based on the manipulation of bones), and various strategies collectively referred to as the mind cure (healing based on intensive prayer and the belief in mind over matter). Others took on greater responsibility for their own health care, learning about their bodies and how best to avoid disease.

The cyclical nature of medical history is evident. Centuries earlier, Hippocrates insisted on treating the whole person—including the mind—and not just malfunctioning bodily parts. The non-traditionalists in the 1800s agreed with this view. In between, minds and bodies were split apart, put back together again, and then split apart once more.

The alternative forms of healing, representing noninvasive approaches to illness, became popular. Much of their strength stemmed from the fact that they offered comprehensive theories of health *and* disease which included an important role for psychological influences. Orthodox medicine focused on disease only. Just as the mind was being linked to the healing of the body, however, history took another turn. Minds and bodies were, one more time, split apart for political and not scientific reasons.

What happened? In response to the Popular Health Movement and the competition presented by unorthodox physicians, traditionalists fought back. One of their first moves was to organize. The American Medical Association, for example, was formed in 1846. This group worked to gain control of hospitals, to enforce a code of ethics that excluded homeopaths from licensure, and to win back the hearts (and pocketbooks) of the general public.[5]

1850–1900 During this period, medical traditionalists regained and solidified their previous status. Around 1860, most conventional physicians stopped treating disease with bleeding and purging, and they replaced obviously dangerous drugs like calomel with "sophisticated" ones like alcohol, morphine, and—somewhat later—cocaine. These drugs did not for the most part affect the underlying causes of disease, but it did not matter. Patients walked into the doctor's office complaining of pain; they left feeling no pain at all. Towards the end of the century, the problem of widespread addiction to prescribed drugs containing opiates was recognized. There was renewed interest in homeopathy, the mind cure, and similar approaches such as Christian Science. But the political clout of traditionalists was great.

Their hand was strengthened by the invention or adaptation for medical use of:

- instruments for visualizing gross anatomical structures (like the ophthalmoscope, laryngoscope, and X-ray)
- microscopes for linking specific diseases with specific germs and tissue changes
- devices for representing bodily functions in graphical or numerical form (like the spirometer, sphygmomanometer, and electrocardiogram)
- tests of body fluids and tissues

These procedures and inventions changed the face of medicine forever by elevating it to an ostensibly exact science. Doctors now had tests and measures that either confirmed their intuitive diagnoses or offered them diagnoses in the first place.

Treatment of diseases and not people was clearly the focus of this era, as exemplified by the popularity of the *germ theory of infectious disease,* accepted as "the" account of disease by physicians and most of the general public as well. Here are the basic assumptions of the germ theory[6]:

- Germs are necessary and sufficient causes of disease.
- For every disease, there is a specific germ.
- Any treatment that removes the germ from the body will cure the disease.
- Any procedure that prevents the germ from entering the body in the first place will prevent the disease.

Illness was seen as a bodily response to a bodily invasion, to be dealt with by physicians on the one hand and public health workers on the other, as we mentioned in Chapter 6.

Certainly attention to the body is not unreasonable when we are grappling with illness. One cannot ignore the strides made by physicians and public health workers armed with the germ theory of disease. The average life expectancy in the Western world took a great leap when medical practice began to take account of this theory.

But the resurrection of Descartes' dualism was an unfortunate consequence. The "logic" is simple. If there are two entirely separate aspects of people, minds and bodies, and if one aspect is unambiguously implicated in disease, then—here is the leap—the other aspect must have nothing to do with it. Psychological influences on physical health and illness can be ignored, as can anything that the individual might do to bolster or promote health, because he after all is just the battleground for the war between physicians and germs.

It is this implication of the germ theory of infectious disease that we argue against. Granted, germs exist and they are important, but they are not necessary and sufficient conditions for disease. Germs *contribute* to illness; they do not *cause* it. As we have said before, we continually harbor all sorts of germs, yet seldom fall ill.

Today, we know that germs are only part of the picture. There are diseases such as cancer or hypertension that are not caused by germs. And even in the case of infectious illnesses, whether or not we fall ill is determined only in part by the intensity of germs. Other factors contribute as well, including psychological states. We believe that people can exert considerable control over their health, by engaging in health-promoting and disease-preventing practices. These are psychological assertions, not biological ones.

Around 1900   Despite the popularity of the germ model, there were further attempts to link minds and bodies. At the turn of the century, Sigmund Freud (1856–1939) began to explain physical ailments in psychological terms. He even went so far as to treat such problems with psychological interventions. Most frequently, his patients had hysteria, a puzzling set of physical losses and disabilities which often beset young women.

Here is Freud's description of a hysterical patient, one Lucy R:

> Lately she complained of some new symptoms. . . . She had totally lost her sense of smell and was almost continuously pursued by one or two subjective olfactory sensations. . . . She was, moreover, in low spirits and fatigued, and she complained of heaviness in the head, diminished appetite, and loss of efficiency.[7]

Freud hypnotized Lucy, as well as his other hysterical patients, and enjoyed much success from this treatment plan.

The history of hysteria is just as bizarre as the range of symptoms that characterized it. Over the centuries, it had been viewed as a female disorder, hence its name (*hysterus* is the Latin word for womb).

Physicians thought that a woman's womb somehow left its proper location and wandered about the body until it lodged someplace else, producing strange symptoms. By the 1900s, the view of hysteria as a wandering womb had died away, but it was still seen as a physical problem, and hence it was appropriately treated with physical means. Freud's psychological approach was notable indeed.

Freud of course went on to propose psychoanalysis: an account of psychopathology and its treatment, normal personality, culture, history, and the arts. However, the psychological explanation of hysteria was yet another failed attempt to join minds with bodies. Why? The symptoms of hysteria came to be seen as not real, at least in a biological sense. To be sure, the hysteric was unable to see or hear or swallow or move, but because there was no physiological cause underlying these symptoms, they were switched from the realm of the body into the realm of the mind. The curious assumptions that legitimized this move were, again, part of our legacy from Descartes.

The 1930s and 1940s   The psychoanalytic tradition informed the development of the field known as psychosomatic medicine, pioneered by Franz Alexander, who viewed various illnesses as physiological reactions to specific psychological states.[8] Part of his explanation satisfied—in principle—the most ardent of the "body" theorists, because he tried to explain the biological pathway from conflicts and emotions to tissue damage.

Suppose someone is always hostile and competitive. He thus experiences chronic excitation of his body's emergency response, a mechanism that readies all of us for fight or flight under threat. According to Alexander, he will develop chronic high blood pressure. Or suppose someone is always passive and dependent. She ends up experiencing chronic inhibition of the emergency response and becomes at risk for a peptic ulcer.

Here are five other illnesses that Alexander theorized about:

• asthma—a fear of separating from mother
• arthritis—inhibited hostility
• colitis—an inability to fulfill obligations
• hyperthyroidism—psychic trauma
• acne—guilt over exhibitionism

Each illness is thought to have a symbolic as well as physiological relationship to an underlying conflict. Alexander's pronouncements were influential for years.

But many have not survived careful scrutiny.[9] His best evidence consisted of striking case examples like the following:

> A young woman for six months began suffering from early ulcerative colitis. Under medical management . . . the bowel had become entirely quiescent. . . . After three months of medical management she complained of a precipitous recurrence of her diarrhea on the preceding Sunday morning. Careful interrogation revealed that she had no undue excitement on the previous Saturday evening. . . . About one hour after breakfast, while she was working around the house, diarrhea appeared. When further questioned on the situations of that Sunday morning when she was at home with her husband, . . . [she] revealed that her husband had asked her, facetiously or otherwise, "What about the $400 I loaned you when we first got married to buy your trousseau? When am I going to get it back?" She didn't have the $400. She felt distinctly disturbed, regressed into a childhood pattern and got diarrhea. When the analyst pointed out to her the association with the money and her inability to give it back except with bowel movements, the condition immediately cleared up.[10]

Earlier, we cautioned against the danger of inferring too much from striking cases (Chapter 2). In this one, we cannot tell which came first—the symptom or the conflict, and whether the patient's insight, achieved in psychotherapy, was *the* curative agent. Indeed, studies with larger numbers of patients that took a more careful look at alternative explanations of results did not for the most part reveal the conflicts that Alexander hypothesized.[11]

The 1950s and 1960s   In 1956, Hans Selye offered an influential description of how the body responded to stress.[12] As we explained in Chapter 3, his work led to many studies of the specific links between stress and illness. Once these were established, other investigators found that unambiguously psychological factors were critical. That is, an event becomes stressful and likely to predispose someone to illness to the degree that he thinks about it in a particular way.

At the same time, a battle began within psychology, one with far-reaching implications for the pertinence of psychological states to health and illness. We are referring to the cognitive revolution. Up until the 1960s, the behaviorists and psychoanalysts—rivals for decades—had carried on their usual academic and intellectual debates. Despite their differences, they had reached a truce of sorts. Behaviorists occupied laboratories; psychoanalysts occupied clinics. And at a certain distance, they could be seen to share a similar view of human nature.

Behaviorists on the one hand saw human beings as passive entities, manipulated by the rewards or punishments offered by their environments. Some will recall the cartoon in which one rat in a maze confides to another, just out of earshot of the experimenter, "Boy, do I have *him* conditioned. Every time I run down the maze, he drops some cheese into it!" It captures the behaviorist view of rats and people alike. Our behaviors are responses to particular environmental stimuli—reactions rather than actions.

Psychoanalysts on the other hand also saw human beings as passive entities shoved around, manipulated not by external rewards and punishments but by internal needs and drives that eluded their awareness. Everything done or not done was in the service of a sexual or aggressive instinct. The entire process took place on an unconscious level.

Although behaviorists located causality outside the person, and the psychoanalysts located it inside, in both cases, the person was never in charge of what he or she did. Thoughts and beliefs could be dismissed as completely irrelevant. People were mindless rather than mindful, senseless rather than sensible.

To understand the reasons for the cognitive revolution, we draw on Howard Gardner's historical account.[13] He felt that several developments converged to bring about reform:

- the availability of new methods to study people's thinking
- the impact of Noam Chomsky's linguistic theories, which showed behaviorist accounts of language to be untenable
- the theories of child psychologist Jean Piaget, who showed that children indeed think differently than adults
- the growing popularity of a cognitive perspective in other social sciences like sociology and anthropology

We add common sense: if we are going to understand what people are all about, at some point we *must* take into account their thoughts and beliefs.

According to Gardner, perhaps the central impetus of the cognitive revolution was the advent of the digital computer. Computers have influenced society as a whole in obvious ways: by allowing massive amounts of information to be stored and manipulated. And they have influenced psychology in particular: by allowing experiments to be automated and data to be rapidly analyzed. But psychologists have found them important for another reason. Computers provide a new and productive model of human nature. Like computers, people take in information, transform it according to rules and strategies, and then behave in accordance with it. Because we perform this so-called information processing, we are seen as intelligent, purposeful, and rational—engaged in the business of making sense of the world.

We indeed behave according to our thoughts and beliefs. If we are wrong, then we try to change our minds in light of what we have learned. If our theories about the world prove useful, allowing us to anticipate and navigate what happens, then we stick with them. In short, the computer metaphor depicts people as engaged in a complex give and take with the environment—a far cry from the behaviorist metaphor of people as stimulus-response units, or the psychoanalytic view of people as wild beasts held in check by a thin tether.

Albert Bandura calls the give and take between people and their environments reciprocal determinism.[14] People influence the world, and the world influences people, back and forth. At the center of reciprocal determinism are cognitions, which allow the individual to make sense of this give and take. In the cognitive revolution, many of the traditional conceptual dichotomies were bridged: thought and action, feeling and thinking, person and environment, and most importantly mind and body.[15] We can now speak of complex belief systems that catalyze our actions and prove sensitive to reality.

The 1970s The new interest in cognition and the pioneering research on stress and coping helped spur the development of a new field, health psychology, within which our work on optimism finds its home. Health psychologists try to determine how people's thoughts, feelings, and actions enter into the equation that describes physical well-being. We may be entering an era where psychologists can be as effective in promoting good health as physicians, because many of the risk factors for contemporary illnesses are psychological in nature. If psychologists can help people to change unhealthy habits or better yet to avoid developing them in the first place, then the health of an entire society can be improved. As we speculated in the last chapter, perhaps clinical psychologists in the next generation will be involved in the treatment of not just anxiety and depression but physical illnesses as well.

The 1980s   This vision is not far-fetched, especially in light of the recent coalescence of yet another field—psychoneuroimmunology—centering on the relationship between the mind and the body's immune system. Although this field is controversial,[16] studies suggest that the central nervous system can directly influence the vigor with which the body defends itself against disease.[17] We described some of this work in Chapter 5.

Other discoveries of psychoneuroimmunologists are also amazing. For example, a research team discovered the hormone ACTH being manufactured in the immune system of human beings.[18] In light of prevailing theories, this did not make sense. It was thought that ACTH was produced in the brain *only,* specifically in the pituitary gland. Yet white blood cells were apparently producing the same hormone as brain cells. To suggest that the mind (brain) and body (immune system) were linked at such a "grass roots" level was to raise a host of questions that scientists are still attempting to answer. Apparently, there is some sort of direct communication going on between the mind and body. But what is being said? How often are they talking to each other? Can we eavesdrop on their conversations, or perhaps even interrupt and somehow speed up (or unblock) the healing process?

What we do know is that the brain and the immune system are in regular biochemical contact. Our defense system against disease is thus akin to a sensory organ: the "eyes" of our body. It senses a virus, for example, and lets the brain in on its discovery, which then spurs the immune system to fight off the virus. And thus the circle is complete: body, mind, body.

In sum   History suggests that we will continue to debate the exact mechanisms linking the mind and the body as well as the reality of the connections. Clearly, money and power are factors in this debate, and as in the nineteenth century, the "mind" proponents may have difficulties with the medical establishment.

At the same time, minds and bodies will probably never be conceptually split as completely as they once were. There is disenchantment with traditional medical conceptions of illness as a problem of the body only.[19] There is renewed interest in alternative medical approaches that take into account the whole person.[20] "Wellness" is becoming a major societal concern.[21] And most importantly, there is a growing body of sound scientific investigations documenting psychological influences on the onset and course of illness.

We do fear a "nothing but" framework that fails to encompass the complexity of health and illness.[22] Psychological states are important, but so too are a host of other influences. We also fear a "blame the victim" mentality in which people who fall ill are held morally responsible for their problems. And we fear disputes within and between the helping professions that are driven by crass concerns. Finally, to use Arthur Barsky's phrase, we fear that people may become "worried sick" about being healthy, precisely because they have not thought enough about what it means to be healthy.[23]

Research definitions of physical health, as discussed in Chapter 2, all seem to boil down to the absence of one or more criteria of illness. But optimal health is not simply the absence of symptoms or illness or high cholesterol counts or abnormal electrocardiograms. Optimal health is a means to an end, and the end is a satisfying life— work and play and friendship and love and family and spiritual experience. One's physical state can make it easy or difficult to attain one's goals, but we question whether the absence of illness should be a goal in its own right.

Optimism and Society

Throughout the book, we have described individuals as optimistic or pessimistic. But *groups* of people can be similarly characterized. Optimism and pessimism are contagious states, meaning that people in the vicinity of one another come to think in similar ways. These ideas lead us to consider how optimism fits within our larger society.

Collective optimism   We will coin the term "collective optimism" to describe the shared beliefs of people in a group that the causes of bad events that befall their group are external and circumscribed. This definition strictly parallels our notion of an individual's optimistic explanatory style. "Collective pessimism" is the group equivalent of an individual's pessimistic explanatory style. Several studies show that collective optimism and pessimism exist and have important consequences for how a group functions.

Gabrielle Oettingen and her colleagues used the CAVE technique we explained in Chapter 1 to ask if cultures differ in their collective optimism or pessimism.[24] They chose for comparison East Berlin and West Berlin. The similarity of the two Berlins with respect to geographical location, language, and history through 1945 makes any differences that might be found more interpretable.

The 1984 Winter Olympics provided the raw material for the CAVE analysis. The games, of course, were extensively covered, and one of the few topics that both East Berlin and West Berlin newspapers described. Oettingen and her colleagues read papers from both sides of the Berlin Wall and extracted events and their causal explanations. When explaining the victories and losses of their own athletes and teams, East Berlin sports stories contained more pessimistic causal explanations than did West Berlin stories about their own athletes and teams.

This difference is striking because East Germany did much better in these games than West Germany, winning 24 medals as opposed to only 4. Regardless, a relatively pessimistic tone permeated the stories read by the East Berliners. A much more extensive study would be needed to know if such stories make the citizens pessimistic, or if pessimistic citizens somehow lead to negative stories. What we can say is that two groups of people indeed differ in their collective optimism and pessimism. We write these paragraphs as thousands of East Berliners are crossing the border to West Berlin. In our view, they are seeking optimism—hope for a better future.

What are the consequences of collective optimism? We hypothesize that collective optimism benefits a group just as individual optimism benefits the single person. In other words, we expect collective optimism to be associated with perseverance, productivity, and good morale. With Julie Jacobs at the University of Michigan, we administered questionnaires to 150 people who were members of groups ranging from social cliques to service organizations to work teams. We asked them about how they saw each group's collective optimism or pessimism, as well as about how the group responded to setbacks and disappointments.

Our results showed that group members do make distinctions with respect to the collective optimism or pessimism of groups and further that the more optimistic groups were those with higher morale, greater cohesiveness, lower turnover of members, and greater willingness to take on new projects and goals. We are currently planning further studies in which we actually observe groups in action, rather than relying on the reports of group members.

Collective optimism and health   The argument advanced in *The Health of Nations,* by epidemiologist Leonard Sagan,[25] is intriguing. Although he does not use the term collective optimism, Sagan theorizes extensively about the notion, linking it explicitly to health. His thesis is that the dramatic increase in people's life expectancy over the last few centuries is *not* the result of medical breakthroughs or public health programs.

Instead, Sagan contends that people live longer nowadays because we have a different psychological makeup. We have become more resilient and more resourceful. We are better educated. We have more meaningful relationships with other people. We have a better articulated sense of self, one characterized by agency and efficacy. These characteristics—which are paraphrased versions of our notion of optimism and its cognates (Chapter 3)—make us healthier people.

Sagan's evidence for this argument is historical. He identifies those periods in which people's life expectancy showed a dramatic jump, and then tries to see what else was going on during these periods. His conclusion is that the jumps do not occur in lockstep with innovations in health practices and services but rather with revisions in how society views the individual. This may be a strange idea if one has not thought about it, but the conception of the "self" indeed varies greatly across historical periods.[26]

In Europe during the Middle Ages, for instances, the idea of individuality as we understand it was for the most part absent. One was born into a role, and one stayed in that role. The same has been true historically in small tribal groups. Expressing oneself, creating an identity, forging a lifestyle, actualizing one's potential, being all that one could be . . . these were not part of the human agenda until relatively recently. Sagan believes that once people started to think of themselves as individual entities with an effect on the world, then people became healthier, and their life expectancy jumped.

Sagan's ideas are extremely controversial, to say the least. But they converge with our conclusions about what happens at the level of individuals. Indeed, individual optimism is legitimized (or not) at the societal level. During its existence, the United States has been an optimistic nation. If and when this societal optimism wanes, then so too will individual optimism. Will the health of our nation take a turn for the worse? Sagan offers the dire prediction that this will happen if Americans become more alienated and disenfranchised than they currently are, despite all the modern medical treatments available now and in the future. Poverty, malnutrition, and the epidemic of drug abuse threaten our nation not just in the obvious biological way, but also psychologically, by undercutting efficacy and resilience.

The very notion of optimism—individual or collective—may be culturally and historically bounded.[27] Although all people have expectations about the future, perhaps the psychological importance of such expectations varies across time and place. Perhaps optimism and pessimism as we have been discussing them are potent psychological dispositions only for residents in Western societies during the late twentieth century.

Among people with a highly articulated sense of self as separate from the world, who exalt individuality and try to "predict and control" the events they encounter, optimism and pessimism should prove critical. But among people with a different psychological makeup, optimism and pessimism may simply be irrelevant to health and illness. By this argument, Sagan's historical analysis is misguided, confusing correlation (between psychological characteristics and longevity) with causation.

Optimism and leadership   In Chapter 6, we concluded that people are attracted to optimistic others. Recent research by Harold Zullow at the University of Pennsylvania suggests that this dynamic is played out not just on an individual level but also on a societal level.[28] He used the CAVE technique to score the optimism or pessimism expressed in the nomination acceptance speeches of presidential candidates from 1948 to 1984. He also ascertained the tendency of these candidates to ruminate, that is, to dwell on bad conditions for themselves or the country.

In these elections—from Dewey versus Truman to Reagan versus Mondale—the eventual winners systematically differed from the eventual losers. Winners were more optimistic in terms of the causal explanations they offered, and they ruminated less. These results held in nine out of ten elections. The only exception was in 1968, where Nixon prevailed over Humphrey despite being slightly more pessimistic. On the other hand, Humphrey brought with him into the campaign the Chicago riots as well as the briefest time interval in recent history between the convention and the election.

These results show that modern Americans favor as their national leader one who expresses optimism for the future—one who minimizes the possibility of a negative future when he mentions bad events, explaining them in a way that allows all of us to maintain positive expectations. We have no way of knowing if our presidents "really" are optimistic or pessimistic, because their speeches may have been written by others; they were certainly edited by others. But the point remains. We do not elect people we actually know as president.

We vote for images, and an optimistic leader has proven highly attractive in recent years.

Zullow took a particularly close look at the 1988 election between Bush and Dukakis.[29] If one were to study only the nomination acceptance speeches made by these two individuals, then Dukakis would be projected as the eventual leader. He was more optimistic and less ruminative than Bush. However, in the course of the subsequent campaign, the expressed optimism of Dukakis steadily eroded, while that of Bush steadily gained. And of course we know what happened. Bush the optimist trounced Dukakis the pessimist.[30]

These findings do relate to collective optimism. Leaders set the tone for a group—in this case, an entire nation—by the optimism or pessimism that they express. Optimism is attractive, and presumably it is contagious. Perhaps charisma is not so mysterious as some would have it. Charisma on the part of a leader may be the ability to infuse his or her group with collective optimism.

Zullow's research was probably no secret to the campaign staffs directing the 1988 election. The results will certainly be considered in future elections, and we wonder just how they will be translated into action. Remember that the optimism which predicts eventual appeal to voters is *not* Pollyannaism. As we have taken pains to make clear, optimism that is too estranged from reality is not true optimism. A casual reading of Zullow's results might suggest to a campaign staff that a candidate should run on outrageous claims.[31] These will of course backfire.

The Future

Many contemporary Americans look healthy and happy on the surface. Recent studies of changes in the incidence of depression over the decades, however, suggest that today's young adults are much more likely to be depressed than their parents or grandparents—perhaps ten times more so![32] Given the strong link between depression and pessimism, we infer that pessimism itself is also becoming more prevalent.

The opposite of collective optimism is collective pessimism, what sociologists for years have been calling alienation. The traditional explanation of alienation is that it occurs in a society in which the relationship between what people do and what then happens to them is obscured: the societal equivalent of a learned helplessness experiment

(Chapter 5). There are other routes to collective pessimism as well, not the least important of which is via the information about the countless hazards to life and happiness with which the general public is bombarded.

Here popular books on personal problems must shoulder part of the blame for the difficulties they purport to solve. In calling people's problems with work, shopping, sexuality, and chocolate "addictions" rather than bad habits, some writers make these more imposing than they need to be.[33] Addiction is an internal, stable, and global explanation for a problem in life; in our terms, it is a pessimistic construal that leads to helplessness and hopelessness.

Further, some popular writers give advice that is too simple to be helpful to any but a handful of people. In a survey of those who relied on typical self-help books, Rosen found scant evidence for their effectiveness in actually solving problems.[34] Large-scale changes in one's lifestyle cannot be accomplished quickly and easily. Those led to believe that they can be are at risk for pessimism, and ultimately helplessness and hopelessness.

On a more optimistic note, we predict that the psychological foundation of health promotion will be strengthened in the future. Psychologists will move into fitness centers and help to devise and implement strategies for achieving health goals.

However, psychological strategies carried out by individuals are just part of the health picture. Although we have not emphasized them in this book, social institutions play an overarching role in making good health more versus less likely.[35] People's status in society influences their exposure to stressful situations as well as how they cope with them. Social support is available to individuals or not depending on their place in the social structure.

When Optimism Is Not Enough

Rothbaum, Weisz, and Snyder chide contemporary psychologists—including us—for focusing unduly on what they call primary control: whether or not people can change actual events in the world.[36] Sometimes primary control is impossible; optimism may be at odds with reality. Some people in difficult circumstances become helpless and hopeless, depressed and ill. Other people continue to cope by accommodating themselves to uncontrollable events.

Primary control represents an attempt to change the *world*. In contrast, accommodating oneself to uncontrollable bad events involves changing the *self*. Rothbaum et al. call the strategies at one's disposal for changing the self secondary control. One such strategy is finding meaning or purpose in otherwise traumatic occurrences. "I learned what was really important in life," say some people after a brush with death.

To the degree that people can make sense of bad events, they can blunt their harmful effects. Numerous philosophies, secular and religious, are available for the purpose of secondary control. We endorse no one philosophy in particular. A person must find one that fits with her own web of belief. But regardless of its content, Rothbaum et al. conclude that such a philosophy is useful.

Sociologist Aaron Antonovsky introduces a similar idea, sense of coherence, which he defines as the ability to find structure, meaning, and regularity in the events that one experiences.[37] Sense of coherence is related to how one copes with demands posed by the world, but it is a broader notion than simply exerting control over outcomes. The person with a sense of coherence regards demands as challenges worthy of attention. Antonovsky argues that sense of coherence is linked to good health, and its absence to poor health.

With Jennifer Bryce, Ned Kirsch, and Kim Lachman, we are in the process of testing some of these hypotheses about the benefits of finding significance in life's traumas. Just as we did for optimism, we developed a questionnaire that measures the degree to which someone tries to find meaning in bad events (see Table 8–1) as well as a content

TABLE 8–1. Items from the Secondary Control Questionnaire

Respondents are asked to indicate their relative agreement or disagreement with statements like these.

1. I take a philosophical approach to what happens to me.
2. What's good or bad depends entirely on your point of view.
3. There are lessons to be learned from every experience.
4. I try to understand the meaning of life.
5. God has a specific plan for me.
6. I'm a believer in the idea that disappointments and setbacks can be good experiences if you learn from them.
7. I adapt myself to what happens.

analysis procedure that can be used to score secondary control (or its absence) from verbal material.

In our first study, we examined the first-person narratives of two groups of people who arguably experienced a great number of uncontrollable life events but nonetheless survived quite well. The first was former American slaves who told their stories to interviewers during the 1930s in conjunction with the Federal Writers Project, a massive undertaking in which survivors of slavery were located and interviewed.[38] At the time they told their stories, the people were elderly. They necessarily had survived the trauma of slavery and its aftermath. By the logic of Rothbaum et al., secondary control strategies should be prominent in their accounts. Here was a group of people for whom primary control was not possible, yet they still coped effectively, as shown by their longevity.

The second was a group of mothers raising their families in the war zone of contemporary Beirut.[39] Again, these people were physically and mentally healthy, despite their lack of control over events happening around them. Again, according to Rothbaum et al., they should be using secondary control strategies.

For comparison purposes, we also looked at first-person narratives from two samples of contemporary Americans: students at an exclusive college and upper middle-class adults. Obviously, these are not ideal comparison groups. They differ from the slaves and the Lebanese mothers in terms of the objective uncontrollability of the events befalling them, but also in other ways.

Regardless, we predicted that the use of secondary control would be more prevalent in the first two samples than in the latter two, by virtue of the greater stress to which these people were exposed and in light of their continued thriving. This pattern is exactly what we found. The former slaves and the mothers in Beirut were much more likely to describe attempts to find meaning in bad events around them than were the American college students and adults. These individuals typically described bad events in terms of their attempts to change them.

We also undertook a more tightly controlled investigation of the mitigating effect of secondary control. Where our first study used a content analysis procedure to search for mention of secondary control, our second investigation used the questionnaire we devised that measures the degree to which a respondent endorses strategies of secondary control.

This questionnaire was administered to a group of students,

along with others assessing explanatory style, stressful life events, and depressive symptoms. We expected an overall correlation between bad events and depression, but we further predicted that the use of secondary control strategies would mitigate this relationship. So, we sought to test the same prediction as in the first study: that secondary control is associated with doing well in the face of bad life events. Again, the results were as predicted. Secondary control reduced the depressing effects of stress. We also found that optimistic explanatory style was associated with less depression in the wake of bad events— *independently* of secondary control.

Thus, two different strategies are associated with robustness in the face of stress. Optimism is one of these. But secondary control— the ability to find meaning in misfortune even when the world itself cannot be changed—is also useful.[40] These strategies are not incompatible. The person who has both available is better able to cope than the person who has but one or neither.

Notes

Chapter 1. Optimism

1. Gay, 1963.
2. Porter, 1913.
3. Porter, 1913, p. 85.
4. Porter, 1913, p. 240.
5. Dakof & Taylor, 1990.
6. Hales & Hales, 1987.
7. Shankland, 1947.
8. Park & Sheff, 1989.
9. Lauzanne & Wylie, 1931.
10. Weston, 1986.
11. Meyer, 1980.
12. Woodruff-Pak, 1988.
13. Lazarus, 1979, 1984.
14. Cf. Engel, 1968; Lefcourt, 1973.
15. Hackett & Cassem, 1974.
16. Taylor & Brown, 1988.
17. Langer, 1978, 1989.
18. E.g., Wong & Weiner, 1981.
19. Nisbett & Wilson, 1977.
20. Heider, 1958; Kelley, 1973; Kelly, 1955; Weiner, 1986.
21. Peterson & Seligman, 1984.
22. Abramson, Seligman, & Teasdale, 1978.
23. Peterson et al., 1982.
24. Peterson, Schulman, Castellon, & Seligman, in press.
25. Peterson & Seligman, 1984.
26. Seligman, 1975.
27. Overmier & Seligman, 1967; Seligman & Maier, 1967.
28. Seligman, Maier, & Peterson, in press.

Chapter 2. Health and Optimism

1. Cousins, 1981.
2. Siegel, 1986, 1989.
3. Cf. Greenwald, 1975.
4. Verbrugge, 1989.
5. The reasons for the sex differences in morbidity and mortality are not at all understood. They may reflect inherent biological differences between the sexes, cultural factors that distinguish between men and women, or some combination of the two.

179

6. Radner, 1989.

7. Vaillant, 1977, p. 3.

8. Vaillant, 1977.

9. Vaillant, 1983.

10. We wish we could reproduce several of these answers in their entirety, but our desire to protect the confidentiality of the participating subjects limits our ability to give a full sense of what and how they wrote.

11. Peterson, Seligman, & Vaillant, 1988.

12. See Vaillant (1977) for more details.

13. Attention in the popular media was overwhelming, and this particular study was featured in articles appearing, among other places, in the *New York Times,* the *Boston Globe, Reader's Digest, Psychology Today, American Health, Muscle and Fitness, Vogue, Better Homes and Gardens, Self, Mature Outlook,* and *Science News.* A representative from Oprah Winfrey's show even called us to discuss optimism, but apparently we weren't sensational enough to warrant further attention. The only call that we did not return was from the *National Enquirer.*

14. Rosenthal & Rubin, 1982.

15. Psychological factors were of course at work earlier, setting the stage for what we later found. Our point is that the effect of optimism on health *as measured here* took years to become evident.

16. Peterson, 1988b.

17. Suls & Mullen, 1981.

18. Costa & McCrae, 1987.

19. Peterson, Colvin, & Lin, 1989.

20. Sears, Maccoby, & Levin, 1957.

21. Levy et al., 1987.

22. Kamen et al., 1987.

23. The immune system is much more complex than our brief description suggests, and there is legitimate debate about how best to interpret such indices as the T4/T8 ratio. Certainly, helper cells and suppressor cells are just two of many interacting "players" on the immunological team. For readable introductions to how the immune system works, see Desowitz (1987) and Jaret (1986).

24. Depression and pessimism are entwined, as we will explain in Chapter 5. However, they are not perfectly redundant, which means it is possible to distinguish their separate effects on health.

25. Schleifer et al., 1985.

26. Burns & Seligman, 1986.

27. Gavzer, 1988.

28. Sontag, 1979, 1988.

29. It is understandable to want to know the reasons for misfortunes, but sometimes there simply is no good explanation. Bad things happen, even to good people, as Harold S. Kushner (1983) reminds us in his best-selling book. An incessant search for why illness and other tragedies occur may only exacerbate one's sorrow.

30. Whether given personality traits characterize people susceptible to various diseases has a long and contested history (e.g., Fox, 1978). However, Hans Eysenck (1988) has recently described two studies of individuals who developed either heart disease or cancer; characteristic premorbid personality styles were evident in both studies. Heart disease was foreshadowed by a style in which the person was exces-

sively emotional and irritable in response to stress. Cancer was foreshadowed by a style marked by helplessness, hopelessness, depression, and inhibition of emotions in the face of stress. Optimism as we see it cuts across these styles, so there is no basis here for arguing that optimism confers a specific immunity to one or the other type of disease (Chapter 5). Regardless, these are exactly the sort of interpretations against which Sontag argues, but facts are facts.

31. Although the *average* life expectancy has steadily increased throughout much of the nineteenth and twentieth centuries, there is no good evidence that the *maximum* life expectancy has changed at all.

32. Consider the notions of Mary Baker Eddy, the founder of Christian Science (Podmore, 1963). On the one hand, we agree with her premise that the mind influences health. On the other hand, Mrs. Eddy went one step beyond this and argued that illness was an illusion. To the true-thinking individual, there is never an illness. "All is mind," went the slogan, although some people are sufficiently confused to believe they have material bodies that fall ill. Even death is an illusion, able to be seen through if one is sufficiently enlightened. However, studies of Christian Scientists suggest that they do *not* live as long as other people, despite the fact that they avoid tobacco and alcohol (e.g., Simpson, 1989).

It may be unfair to criticize Mrs. Eddy's beliefs on scientific grounds, in that her approach was ostensibly religious. However, she is the one who added "science" to the title, meaning precisely that this belief system was to be evaluated on such grounds. We find it lacking. Indeed, as other critics have pointed out, Christian Science initially flourished precisely among those who were in a position to pretend that physical reality didn't impinge on health. Its practitioners were already healthy and affluent, sheltered and well-fed.

33. This goes by different names in different psychotherapies, but it seems to be a pervasive practice. Psychoanalysts call it working through the transference, behavior modifiers call it counterconditioning, client-centered therapists see it as providing an atmosphere of unconditional acceptance, and cognitive therapists (Chapter 7) see it as combating one's automatic thoughts. Regardless, the intent is to throw off the influence of the past so that the future will be different.

Chapter 3. Positive Thoughts and Good Health

1. Scheier & Carver, 1985.
2. Scheier & Carver, 1985, 1987.
3. Scheier et al., 1989.
4. Kobasa, 1979.
5. Kobasa, Maddi, & Courington, 1981.
6. Kobasa, 1979.
7. Kobasa, 1982.
8. Kobasa, Maddi, & Kahn, 1982.
9. Bandura, 1977, 1986.
10. O'Leary, 1985, pp. 448–449.
11. Peterson & Stunkard, 1989.
12. Bandura et al., 1985.
13. Bandura, 1987.
14. Bandura, 1986.

15. Cobb, 1976.

16. Tillmann & Hobbs, 1949.

17. Cohen & Syme, 1985.

18. House et al., 1982.

19. Among women in the sample, there was not such a marked difference in mortality between those who did versus did not perform regular volunteer work, although the relationship was still in the same direction as the men. Perhaps typical women already are so busy taking care of other people that "official" volunteer work does not so dramatically bolster their health.

20. Pennebaker & O'Heeron, 1984.

21. Pennebaker, Hughes, & O'Heeron, 1987.

22. Comstock & Partridge, 1972.

23. Obviously, not *all* social support is as helpful as we have been stating. Sometimes it is irrelevant, the wrong sort at the wrong time. Sometimes it undercuts people's sense of their own abilities to solve things. Sometimes it makes a person feel badly because it contradicts her particular thoughts and feelings. Remember the example in Chapter 1 of how pie-in-the-sky optimism makes seriously ill individuals feel inhibited and even resentful, because they cannot express their "negative" thoughts and feelings.

24. Selye, 1956.

25. Rabkin & Struening, 1976.

26. Holmes & Rahe, 1967.

27. Kanner, Coyne, Schaefer, & Lazarus, 1981.

28. Weinberger, Hiner, & Tierney, 1987.

29. In *Healthy Work,* Karasek and Theorell (1990) described how the various factors that exacerbate stress can come together in the workplace to threaten health. The most stressful jobs are those that combine high pressure to perform with little decision latitude. Bosses thus have fewer stress-related illnesses than do their employees. These findings have an ominous implication for women entering the work force, because they are more likely than men to be given stressful jobs, such as operating computerized equipment in an automated office.

30. Lazarus, 1966, 1982; Lazarus & Folkman, 1984.

31. McClelland, 1989.

32. Friedman & Rosenman, 1974.

33. Glass, 1977.

34. Early studies documented the link between Type A behavior and heart attacks. More recent investigations have not been as successful in showing this link (e.g., Ragland & Brand, 1988b), which raises intriguing questions. Were the early studies somehow flukes? Or has the link between Type A behavior and cardiac problems actually changed over time, perhaps because of widespread publicity? Fearing a heart attack, some Type A individuals may intentionally modify not their style, but their diet and level of exercise.

35. Matthews, 1982.

36. Van Egeren, 1979.

37. Matthews, 1982.

38. E.g., Krantz, Glass, & Snyder, 1974.

39. Brunson & Matthews, 1981.

40. Weidner and Andrews (1983), using a questionnaire very similar to the ASQ,

did find a relationship between pessimistic explanatory style and Type A behavior. Similarly, Scheier and Carver (1987) reported a moderate relationship between pessimism as measured on the LOT and the Type A tendency.

41. An opposite phenomenon—the postponement of death until after important occasions—has also been validated in recent research. Phillips and Smith (1990) found that mortality rates among Chinese-Americans in California showed a consistent dip the week before the Harvest Moon Festival and a consistent peak the week following.

42. Stroebe & Stroebe, 1987.

43. Stroebe & Stroebe, 1987, p. 167.

44. Wortman & Silver, 1989. These researchers have also shown that myths to the contrary, there is no "standard" pattern to grief. Mourners display considerable variation, and no one approach to grief can be described as the most healthy. Those who do not mourn openly should not be accused of denial; those who take a long time to finish mourning should not be accused of self-indulgence.

45. Tolle et al., 1986.

46. Gibbs, 1989.

47. Stroebe & Stroebe, 1983.

48. E.g., Bartrop et al., 1977.

49. Ornstein & Sobel, 1984, 1989; Justice, 1988; Locke & Colligan, 1986.

50. Peirce, 1955.

51. Cassileth et al., 1985.

52. Case et al., 1985.

53. A recently reported study suggests that the relationship between Type A behavior pattern and heart attacks following an initial one is quite complex (Ragland & Brand, 1988a). Whereas Type As are more likely than Type Bs to have a first attack, they may be less likely to have a second one. The exact reason for this is not clear. Perhaps Type As have more severe heart attacks in the first place and thus tend not to live long enough to have a second one; perhaps not.

54. Case et al., 1985, p. 740.

55. Angell, 1985a.

56. Angell, 1985a, p. 1571.

57. Angell, 1985a, p. 1571.

58. Abeles, 1986.

59. Angell, 1985b.

Chapter 4. The Origins of Optimism

1. Piaget, 1926, 1928, 1929, 1932, 1950.

2. Watson, 1977.

3. Fincham & Cain, 1986.

4. McLeod, 1987.

5. Brown & Harris, 1978.

6. Dweck, 1975.

7. Bandura, 1986.

8. This point is analogous to the one made in Chapter 2: it may take years for the effects of optimism or pessimism to show a measurable effect on health, but this does not mean that they are dormant within the person until this time.

9. Dweck & Elliot, 1983.

10. Parsons & Ruble, 1977.

11. Weisz, 1983.

12. Ruble, Parsons, & Ross, 1976.

13. Nicholls, 1979; Stipek, 1981.

14. Nolen-Hoeksema, 1986.

15. Dean, Klavens, & Peterson, 1989.

16. Bower, 1981.

17. E.g., Jaynes & Williams, 1989.

18. Remember in Chapter 3 that church attendance is associated with better health, presumably because it brings people into supportive contacts with others. The present finding introduces a subtlety: religiosity on the part of one's parents may not lead a child to grow up to be optimistic. We wish we had asked more questions in this section, particularly about church attendance and participation in church activities.

19. Among adults, there is an attributional tradeoff between ability and effort in terms of its perceived effect on their achievement. The same performance is due either to ability or to hard work—not both. If someone works hard, it is inferred that he or she lacks ability. Those who have ability are assumed not to work as hard. We do not endorse these beliefs, and we are skeptical that they reflect the way achievement actually works. But this is how many adults tend to see matters.

20. Sears, Maccoby, & Levin, 1957.

21. This is the same sample on which we replicated the optimism-health link (p. 35 in Chapter 2).

22. In other words, granted that a parent institutes overly early bowel training—at odds with the neurological capabilities of an infant—what else does this parent do that might adversely affect the development of optimism? Psychiatrists working in a Veterans Hospital told us the following story: A young soldier had a severe breakdown shortly after enlisting; per regular procedures, he was discharged from the service and sent to a Veterans Hospital near his home town. His therapists there contacted his mother, and conducted a standard interview with her, asking about notable events in the young man's childhood. Was he breast-fed? Yes. And when was he weaned? His mother was not exactly sure, but she replied that it was at least a few years before he entered the service!?! Did breast feeding into adolescence create his mental difficulties? In and of itself, probably not, but what else was going on in this family granted this unusual event?

23. Seligman, Peterson, et al., 1984.

24. We have made this comment repeatedly in the chapter. In there any sign that this pattern will change? For all the rhetoric about changing sex roles in the American family, the fact remains that women still spend more time raising children than men (Bee, 1987). Their "liberation" means going off to work, and is apparently not matched by an increased tendency on the part of their husbands to stay home with the kids.

25. Nolen-Hoeksema, 1986.

26. Vanden Belt, 1989.

27. Peterson, 1988a.

28. E.g., Bibace & Walsh, 1981; Blos, 1978; Burbach & Peterson, 1986; Gochman, 1988; Kalnins & Love, 1982.

29. Wilkinson, 1988.

30. We chuckle, but then we stop and realize that this way of thinking may persist into adolescence. To the childish thinker, safe sex may entail "passing on" as rapidly as possible any sexual contact.

31. Natapoff, 1982, p. 134.

Chapter 5. From Optimism to Health: Biological and Emotional Routes

1. Peterson & Stunkard, 1989.

2. Cf. Barsky, 1988.

3. We believe that most of the general public is aware of this bidirectional influence. We are not so convinced that health promotion "experts" appreciate the point.

4. This "other topic" they were studying was the relationship between two basic types of learning: classical conditioning and operant conditioning. Classical conditioning is the type of learning first described by Pavlov (of the salivating dogs) and was presumably occurring when the dog was placed in the harness and given the original shocks. Operant conditioning is the type of learning of interest to Skinner (of the pecking pigeons) and would presumably show up when the dog was placed in the shuttle box.

5. Overmier & Seligman, 1967; Seligman & Maier, 1967.

6. Maier & Seligman, 1976.

7. Maier, 1970.

8. Peterson & Seligman, 1984.

9. Seligman, 1975, p. 99.

10. Langer, 1975; Wortman, 1975.

11. Peterson & Bossio, 1989.

12. Seligman, Maier, & Peterson, in press.

13. Bandura, 1986.

14. Levine, 1977.

15. Gamzu, 1974.

16. Maier & Jackson, 1979.

17. Maier, Laudenslager, & Ryan, 1985.

18. This is just speculation, but we can use this fact to make sense of an interesting difference in survival times of two groups of people who may have AIDS: homosexual men who contracted the disease through sex and intravenous drug users who contracted the disease through needle-sharing. The homosexuals outlive the narcotics addicts, and perhaps the difference lies in the robustness of their respective immune systems. In the latter case, immune functioning has been severely compromised by the introduction into the body of substances that lodge in the immune system.

19. Kiecolt-Glaser & Glaser, 1987.

20. Suls & Mullen, 1981.

21. Melnechuk, 1985.

22. van Doornen & van Blokland, 1987.

23. Then again, maybe this pathway has nothing to do with biology. It is speculated that testosterone is linked to aggression and aggressiveness, to risk taking, to impulsivity, and the like. As we will explain, perhaps these styles of behaving in turn affect health and illness, not because of the hormones per se but because of the effect of hormones on behaviors.

24. Sweeney, Anderson, & Bailey, 1986.

25. E.g., Schleifer et al., 1985.

26. American Psychiatric Association, 1987, p. 222.

27. Seligman, 1973.

28. Nolen-Hoeksema, 1987.

29. Beck, 1967, 1976.

30. Burns, 1980.

31. Seligman, 1974.

32. The use of so-called analogue research is common in the field of science, although laboratory models are most frequently used to study biochemical and physiological processes, as well as the effects of cosmetics. One of the largest consumers of laboratory animals, specifically rabbits, is the cosmetic industry, which uses rabbits to test the consequences of mascara in human eyes because rabbit eyes and people eyes are similarly irritated. We advise you not to wear eye makeup if you are attending the local animal rights meeting. Less common is the use of a laboratory model to study a psychological process, but learned helplessness research as conducted by Seligman provides an excellent example of how to proceed.

33. Beck, Kovacs, & Weissman, 1975.

34. Bipolar disorder, as we have said, is marked by an alternation of depressive episodes with manic episodes. In many ways, a manic episode shows itself in terms of the opposite symptoms of a depressive episode: increased energy, decreased need for sleep, increased sex drive, thoughts racing, and—of interest for the present purposes—a grandiose sense of self. In other words, a manic individual is inappropriately optimistic. One of us (CP) once worked as a therapist for a manic individual, who was on the verge of moving to Hawaii to take Tom Selleck's place on "Magnum, PI," so convinced was he of his sex appeal. The fact that he looked more like Mr. Magoo than Tom Selleck dissuaded him not a bit. We have no trouble accommodating this in our view of true optimism as realistic, because here the individual moves beyond the limitations of reality.

And what is the relationship between mania and health? This is an interesting question, but it proves difficult to answer because there are few cases of pure mania. We do know about individuals with bipolar disorder. These folks are at increased risk of death—as are those with unipolar depression—by illness, accident, and suicide (e.g., Black, Warrack, & Winokur, 1985).

A recent study by Kronfol and House (1988) found that people's immune functioning was suppressed during manic episodes, just as it is during depressive episodes. This is interesting, yet another reminder that inappropriate optimism is *not* healthy.

35. Egeland et al., 1987.

36. See Gallagher, 1988.

37. Friedman & Booth-Kewley, 1987, p. 552.

38. Norem & Cantor, 1986.

39. Costa & McCrae, 1987.

40. Kaplan & Camacho, 1983; Mossey & Shapiro, 1982.

Chapter 6. From Optimism to Health: Behavioral and Interpersonal Routes

1. Alloy, Peterson, Abramson, & Seligman, 1984.

2. E.g., Diener & Dweck, 1978; Dweck, 1975; Dweck & Reppucci, 1973.

3. *The Sporting News,* June 19, 1989, p. 28.

4. Peterson & Barrett, 1987.

5. Smith, Peterson, & Pintrich, 1989.

6. There is a growing impatience among professionals and the general public alike with the tyranny of typical conceptions of intelligence, particularly the notion that intelligence is but one thing that is biologically rooted. More contemporary statements regard intelligence as plural, and as something that must be examined in the context in which it is used (e.g., Gardner, 1983; Sternberg, 1985). We think these attributes of how optimistic students approach their schoolwork are exactly what an expanded conception of intelligence calls for.

7. Atlas & Peterson, 1989.

8. McCormick & Taber, 1988.

9. The previous example of Pete Rose, ballplayer and gambler, should not be confused with the implications of our racetrack study. In Chapter 1, we cautioned that optimism may differ across domains of life. Rose the ballplayer is a good example of an optimist; we doubt that Rose the gambler so qualifies. On the other hand, nothing we read about his scandal suggested that he lost the baseball bets he made.

10. One use of a negative goal is to combat perfectionism, which we regard as a disguised version of pessimism. Think about it: the perfectionist never believes that anything is good enough and always wants to tinker and meddle some more. If this is not pessimism, what is? But sometimes the perfectionist/pessimist can be encouraged to relinquish a project by instructing him to produce a "bad" version of it. In teaching, one of us (CP) has found it useful to ask students to write—and we quote—"incredibly rough drafts" of papers. The stated rationale is to allow the instructor some input into the process; if the paper is too polished, he is cheated out of the privilege of being able to help with advice. This is true as far as it goes, but unsaid is that a bad draft is better than no draft, representing as it does a sure-fire cure for perfectionism.

11. Peterson & Barrett, 1987.

12. Locke et al., 1981.

13. Bandura, 1977.

14. Seligman & Schulman, 1986.

15. Peterson, Colvin, & Lin, 1989.

16. Alexander, 1988.

17. Seligman, Nolen-Hoeksema, Thornton, & Thornton, 1989.

18. Peterson, 1988b.

19. Belloc, 1973; Belloc & Breslow, 1972.

20. Prochaska et al., 1988.

21. Peterson, Colvin, & Lin, 1989.

22. Lin & Peterson, 1989.

23. Lazarus & Folkman, 1984.

24. This measure was not the Attributional Style Questionnaire, which we would have preferred but sacrificed for the sake of brevity. Instead, subjects responded to a number of questions asking about their expectations regarding their health in the future, and these were readily identifiable as optimistic versus pessimistic (Ditto & Cantor, 1989).

25. Taylor, Denham, & Ureda, 1982.

26. Peterson & Stunkard, 1989.

27. Cobb, 1976.

28. House et al., 1988.

29. Friedmann et al., 1980.
30. E.g., Anderson & Arnoult, 1985.
31. Gotlib & Beatty, 1985.
32. Seligman, Peterson, et al., 1984.
33. Peterson, Colvin, & Lin, 1989.
34. Buss & Craik, 1984.

35. Yet another piece of this picture is provided in a recent study by Scott Bunce (1989) at the University of Michigan, who administered the ASQ to a group of research subjects along with a standard personality inventory that assesses an appreciable range of personality characteristics. His results reveal a very stark contrast between optimists and pessimists with respect to personality traits showing interpersonal presence and facility. Optimists are dominant, extraverted, and confident. Pessimists are shrinking, retiring, submissive wimps. So much for the supposed sophistication of the cynic and the skeptic!

Chapter 7. Becoming an Optimist

1. Quine & Ullian, 1978.
2. Peterson, 1982.
3. Abelson et al., 1968.
4. Mischel, Ebbesen, & Zeiss, 1973.
5. Rokeach, 1971.
6. Ollendick, 1986.
7. Bandura, 1986.
8. King, Hamilton, & Murphy, 1983.
9. Miller, 1983.
10. Ellis, 1962.
11. Shilling, 1984.
12. Beck, 1976; Beck & Emery, 1985; Beck, Rush, Shaw, & Emery, 1979.
13. Hollon & Beck, 1986.
14. Reifman & Peterson, 1989.

15. The good news, of course, is that the Orioles' pessimistic funk was not a permanent one. The following season, the Orioles did a turnabout and played very good baseball. Informal observations of the sports pages show a much more upbeat approach on the part of the players and coaches. What was responsible for the change, not only in performance but in optimism? It may have something to do with the fact that baseball has seasons, which allows a player (or fan) to "compartmentalize" bad events and put them in the past. That was then, this is now. Wait until next year.

16. Peterson & Rosenwald, 1987.
17. Lachman, 1988.
18. Lachman, 1989.
19. Skinner, 1983, p. 24.
20. Seligman et al., 1988.
21. Beck, 1967, 1976.
22. Cook & Peterson, 1986.

23. We are not alone in wondering how *changes* in a person's psychological characteristics end up influencing health. We know from epidemiological studies that

a number of psychological factors are linked to poor health (Chapter 3); we do not yet know if changing these factors can produce good health. The line of work that is furthest along looks at Type A coronary-prone behavior pattern. So far, we know that it can be changed through counseling, and there is tentative evidence that the likelihood of coronary heart disease is thereby decreased (Friedman et al., 1984; Gill et al., 1985). Results will become more clear as time passes.

A recent study has shown that psychotherapy greatly increased the survival time of women with metastatic breast cancer (Spiegel et al., 1989). Compared to otherwise identical patients, women who participated in group therapy once a week for a year lived almost twice as long: 36 months versus 19 months. Therapy sessions focused on how best to cope with cancer and the side effects of its medical treatment. The patients expressed their feelings and encouraged each other to be more assertive with their physicians. The beneficial effects of therapy on survival were not immediately evident. Differences between patients who did and did not have therapy were first evident at eight months following the end of therapy.

The investigators tentatively concluded that the social support that the therapy group provided may have been the crucial ingredient, but they not surprisingly called for future studies. Regardless, their investigation has already attracted a great deal of attention for showing that a psychological intervention can meaningfully improve a patient's health.

24. We hesitated some in deciding whether to make this list of do's and don't's. We wanted to avoid aphorisms, and we did not want this to be a "how-to" book. The steps we sketch are only guidelines; personal details must be filled in so they make most sense to the person who wants to follow them.

25. Berne, 1964.

26. In his fixed-role therapy, psychologist George Kelly (1955) devised a way to change a client's characteristic beliefs. Here is how it works. The therapist devises roles for her client that embody a set of interpretations different than those the client habitually uses. He than takes on the roles and, if all goes smoothly, eventually the worldviews they reflect. Fixed-role therapy is based on Kelly's notion that people have problems because their interpretations of the world produce difficulties for them, a cognitive perspective with which we fully agree.

27. Barsky, 1988.

28. Ornstein & Sobel, 1989.

29. Peterson & Stunkard, 1989.

30. Indeed there is reason to believe that health promotion programs fail to work precisely with individuals and groups that can be termed pessimistic (see Peterson & Stunkard, 1989).

Chapter 8. Taking Stock

1. Williams, 1967.

2. Podmore, 1963.

3. Weil, 1988, p. 13.

4. We can certainly criticize the techniques of heroic medicine, but let us appreciate that traditional physicians were sincere in their attempts to help patients. They were victims of theories that were grievously wrong. So, it was widely believed among doctors that there really was but one disease state, that resulted from an imbalance of

the body's humours (fluids). Depending on the nature of the imbalance, a person developed different symptoms. Further, disease was thought *not* to be self-limiting. Someone who became ill was bound to die unless heroic measures were taken. The idea that the body could heal itself was explicitly disavowed, even mistrusted as mystical (Duffy, 1979).

5. Coulter, 1982.
6. Maher & Maher, 1979.
7. Freud, 1893, pp. 106–107.
8. Alexander, 1939, 1950.
9. Weiner, 1977.
10. Alexander, 1950, pp. 124–125, citing Portis, 1949.
11. One place where Alexander was on target was his hypothesis that hostility and competitiveness were linked to heart disease. This is the same formula captured by the contemporary notion of the Type A coronary-prone behavior pattern, as discussed in Chapter 3.
12. Selye, 1956.
13. Gardner, 1985.
14. Bandura, 1986.
15. The cognitive approach has gained such power that it subsumed the perspectives that it originally opposed—behaviorism and psychoanalysis. Behaviorists have begun to merge their ideas with those of cognitive theorists (e.g., Mahoney, 1974; Meichenbaum, 1977; Mischel, 1979), and psychoanalysts have followed suit (e.g., Colby & Stoller, 1988; Erdelyi, 1985). We would say the cognitive revolution is officially over. Among the benefits that have followed is a sophisticated conception of optimism.
16. Pelletier & Herzing, 1988.
17. Ader & Cohen, 1981.
18. Smith et al., 1986.
19. Siegel, 1986, 1989.
20. Weil, 1988.
21. Yankelovich & Gurin, 1989.
22. The New Age movement is a case in point (Fuller, 1989; Gordon, 1988). On the one hand, New Age individuals embrace some very reasonable notions about the mutual influence of mind and body, wellness, and health promotion. On the other hand, they embrace with equal fervor ideas on the fringe and beyond, like pyramid power, healing crystals, white magic, reincarnation, channeling, and extraterrestials. Certainly, the spiritual aspect of life has been neglected in many American quarters during recent decades, but in what we take to be a reaction to this neglect, the New Age movement goes too far and adopts a "nothing but" approach to the human condition. Here we see a focus on the supernatural world to the exclusion of the natural one. New Age individuals seem to like our research on optimism and health, and favorable mention of our work has appeared in some New Age magazines. We are pleased with the interest, to be sure, but we stress here that our message about health is a mundane one.
23. Barsky, 1988.
24. Oettingen et al., 1988.
25. Sagan, 1987.
26. E.g., Baumeister, 1986; Berger & Luckmann, 1966.

27. Peterson, 1991.

28. Zullow et al., 1988.

29. Zullow, 1988.

30. We cannot help but tweak George Bush, optimistic campaigner *and* law-and-order president, by describing a study we recently completed with Michelle Dean. How does an individual's optimism relate to his or her attitudes toward crime? We administered Scheier and Carver's dispositional optimism measure, discussed in Chapter 3, to 62 adults, along with several measures of their attitudes toward crime and punishment (Dean & Peterson, 1989).

Results reveal that optimists are kinder and gentler than pessimists when it comes to crime and punishment. They believe that the causes of crime are to be found in economic conditions within society, *not* in the makeup of individual criminals. They believe that the purpose of the penal system is to rehabilitate those convicted of crimes, *not* to punish them. They favor parole for those in prison. And they believe that criminals will not repeat their crimes.

31. In a deliberately funny essay, James Gorman (1989) shows how our points can be misinterpreted. He discusses our research program under the rubric "Night of the Living Optimists," suggesting that the real world would become a horror movie if and when the "optimists" took over. Why? Optimists *do* things, whereas pessimists do not. And most of the things done in the world are for the worse, Gorman reasons, so isn't paralysis better than action? He concludes that pessimism is our only hope for the future. Gorman's purpose was humor. But who knows what we will see in the 1992 election, when other purposes will prevail?

32. Seligman, 1988.

33. Addiction proves a difficult to define concept even when applied narrowly to problems with alcohol and drugs (Peele, 1989). Historically, people were considered to be addicted to a substance if they were physically dependent upon it, showing tolerance following increased use and withdrawal following decreased use. But this definition rested on the ability to distinguish physical dependence from psychological dependence, and we know this is difficult if not downright impossible. Many mental health professionals today speak no longer of addiction to drugs but instead of their abuse. Some popular authors have not been so cautious with the concept of addiction, extending it widely, even including other people as addictions.

34. Rosen, 1987.

35. Pearlin, 1989.

36. Rothbaum, Weisz, & Snyder, 1982.

37. Antonovsky, 1987.

38. Yetman, 1970.

39. Bryce, 1986.

40. In Chapter 3, we suggested that a person's incessant search for *why* a misfortune occurred is not always healthy, psychologically or physically. Sometimes wisdom must take the form of knowing when to give up attempts at explaining the twists and turns of life. As the noted philosopher Kenny Rogers once observed, one has to know when to hold cards and know when to fold them.

References

Abeles, N. (1986). Proceedings of the American Psychological Association, Incorporated, for the year 1985: Minutes of the Annual Meeting of the Council of Representatives. *American Psychologist, 41,* 633–663.

Abelson, R. P., Aronson, E., McGuire, W. J., Newcomb, T. M., Rosenberg, M. J., & Tannenbaum, P. H. (1968). *Theories of cognitive consistency: A sourcebook.* Chicago: Rand McNally.

Abramson, L. Y., Seligman, M. E. P., & Teasdale, J. D. (1978). Learned helplessness in humans: Critique and reformulation. *Journal of Abnormal Psychology, 87,* 49–74.

Ader, R., & Cohen, N. (1981). Conditioned immunopharmacological responses. In R. Ader (Ed.), *Psychoneuroimmunology.* New York: Academic Press.

Alexander, F. (1939). Emotional factors in essential hypertension. *Psychosomatic Medicine, 1,* 139–152.

Alexander, F. (1950). *Psychosomatic medicine: Its principles and applications.* New York: Norton.

Alexander, M. (1988). *The effects on caretakers of caring for a head injured relative.* Unpublished doctoral dissertation, University of Michigan.

Alloy, L. B., Peterson, C., Abramson, L. Y., & Seligman, M. E. P. (1984). Attributional style and the generality of learned helplessness. *Journal of Personality and Social Psychology, 46,* 681–687.

American Psychiatric Association (1987). *Diagnostic and statistical manual of mental disorders* (3rd ed., Rev.). Washington, DC: author.

Anderson, C. A., & Arnoult, L. H. (1985). Attributional style and everyday problems in living: Depression, loneliness, and shyness. *Social Cognition, 3,* 16–35.

Angell, M. (1985a). Disease as a reflection of the psyche. *The New England Journal of Medicine, 312,* 1570–1572.

Angell, M. (1985b). [Letter to the editor.] *The New England Journal of Medicine, 313,* 1358–1359.

Antonovsky, A. (1987). *Unraveling the mystery of health: How people manage stress and stay well.* San Francisco: Jossey-Bass.

Atlas, G. D., & Peterson, C. (1989). *Explanatory style among harness racing bettors.* Unpublished manuscript, University of Michigan.

Bandura, A. (1977). Self-efficacy: Toward a unifying theory of behavioral change. *Psychological Review, 84,* 191–215.

Bandura, A. (1986). *Social foundations of thought and action.* Englewood Cliffs, NJ: Prentice-Hall.

Bandura, A. (1987). *Perceived self-efficacy in the exercise of control over AIDS infection.* Paper presented at the National Institutes of Mental Health and Drug Abuse Research Conference on Women and AIDS, Bethesda, MD.

194   References

Bandura, A., Taylor, C. B., Williams, S. L., Mefford, I. N., & Barchas, J. D. (1985). Catecholamine secretion as a function of perceived coping self-efficacy. *Journal of Consulting and Clinical Psychology, 53,* 406–414.

Barsky, A. J. (1988). *Worried sick: Our troubled quest for wellness.* Boston: Little, Brown.

Bartrop, R. W., Luckhurts, E., Lazarus, L., Kiloh, L. G., & Penny, R. (1977). Depressed lymphocyte function after bereavement. *Lancet, 97,* 834–836.

Baumeister, R. F. (1986). *Identity: Cultural change and the struggle for self.* New York: Oxford University Press.

Beck, A. T. (1967). *Depression: Clinical, experimental, and theoretical aspects.* New York: Hoeber.

Beck, A. T. (1976). *Cognitive therapy and the emotional disorders.* New York: International Universities Press.

Beck, A. T., & Emery, G. (1985). *Anxiety disorders and phobias: A cognitive perspective.* New York: Basic Books.

Beck, A. T., Kovacs, M., & Weissman, A. (1975). Hopelessness and suicidal behavior: An overview. *JAMA, 234,* 1146–1149.

Beck, A. T., Rush, A. J., Shaw, B. F., & Emery, G. (1979). *Cognitive therapy of depression.* New York: Guilford.

Bee, H. L. (1987). *The journey of adulthood.* New York: Macmillan.

Belloc, N. B. (1973). Relationship of health practices and mortality. *Preventive Medicine, 2,* 67–81.

Belloc, N. V., & Breslow, L. (1972). Relationship of physical health status and family practices. *Preventive Medicine, 1,* 409–421.

Berger, P. L., & Luckmann, T. (1966). *The social construction of reality.* New York: Doubleday.

Berne, E. (1964). *Games people play.* New York: Grove Press.

Bibace, R., & Walsh, M. E. (Eds.). (1981). *Children's conceptions of health, illness, and bodily functions.* San Francisco: Jossey-Bass.

Black, D. W., Warrack, G., & Winokur, G. (1985). Excess mortality among psychiatric patients: The Iowa Record-Linkage Study. *JAMA, 253,* 58–61.

Blos, P. (1978). Children think about illness: Their concepts and beliefs. In E. Gellert (Ed.), *Psychosocial aspects of pediatric care.* Orlando, FL: Grune & Stratton.

Bower, G. H. (1981). Mood and memory. *American Psychologist, 36,* 129–148.

Brown, G. W., & Harris, T. O. (1978). *Social origins of depression.* New York: Free Press.

Brunson, B. I., & Matthews, K. A. (1981). The Type A coronary-prone behavior pattern and reactions to uncontrollable events: An analysis of learned helplessness. *Journal of Personality and Social Psychology, 40,* 906–918.

Bryce, J. W. (1986). *Cries of children in Lebanon as voiced by their mothers.* Beirut: Express International.

Bunce, S. (1989). *Explanatory style as a trait.* Unpublished masters thesis, University of Michigan.

Burbach, D. J., & Peterson, L. (1986). Children's concepts of physical illness: A review and critique of the cognitive-developmental literature. *Health Psychology, 5,* 307–325.

Burns, D. D. (1980). *Feeling good: The new mood therapy.* New York: Signet.

Burns, M. O., & Seligman, M. E. P. (1986). [Explanatory style and illness measured by elevated temperature.] Unpublished data, University of Pennsylvania.

Buss, D. M., & Craik, K. H. (1984). Acts, dispositions, and personality. In B. A. Maher (Ed.), *Progress in experimental personality research* (Vol. 13). New York: Academic Press.

Case, R. B., Heller, S. S., Case, N. B., Moss, A. J., & The Multicenter Post-Infarction Research Group. (1985). Type A behavior and survival after acute myocardial infarction. *The New England Journal of Medicine, 312,* 737–741.

Cassileth, B. R., Lusk, E. J., Miller, D. S., Brown, L. L., & Miller, C. (1985). Psychosocial correlates of survival in advanced malignant disease? *The New England Journal of Medicine, 312,* 1551–1555.

Cobb, S. (1976). Social support as a moderator of life stress. *Psychosomatic Medicine, 38,* 300–314.

Cohen, S., & Syme, S. L. (1985). *Social support and health.* Orlando, FL: Academic Press.

Colby, K. M., & Stoller, R. J. (1988). *Cognitive science and psychoanalysis.* Hillsdale, NJ: Erlbaum.

Comstock, G. W., & Partridge, K. B. (1972). Church attendance and health. *Journal of Chronic Diseases, 25,* 665–672.

Cook, M. L., & Peterson, C. (1986). Depressive irrationality. *Cognitive Therapy and Research, 10,* 293–298.

Costa, P. T., & McCrae, R. R. (1987). Neuroticism, somatic complaints, and disease: Is the bark worse than the bite? *Journal of Personality, 55,* 299–316.

Coulter, H. L. (1982). *Divided legacy: The conflict between homoeopathy and the American Medical Association.* Berkeley, CA: North Atlantic Books.

Cousins, N. (1981). *The anatomy of an illness.* New York: Norton.

Dakof, G. A., & Taylor, S. E. (1990). Victims' perceptions of social support: What is helpful from whom? *Journal of Personality and Social Psychology, 58,* 80–89.

Dean, M., Klavens, B., & Peterson, C. (1989). [The origins of optimism.] Unpublished data, University of Michigan.

Dean, M., & Peterson, C. (1989). [Optimism and legal attitudes.] Unpublished data, University of Michigan.

Desowitz, R. S. (1987). *The thorn in the starfish: The immune system and how it works.* New York: Norton.

Diener, C. I., & Dweck, C. S. (1978). An analysis of learned helplessness: Continuous changes in performance, strategy, and achievement cognitions following failure. *Journal of Personality and Social Psychology, 36,* 451–462.

Ditto, P. H., & Cantor, N. (1989). *Two faces of optimism: The role of outcome expectancies and intuitive theories of illness in preventive and reactive health behavior.* Paper presented at the Annual Meeting of the Midwestern Psychological Association, Chicago.

Duffy, J. (1979). *The healers: A history of American medicine.* Urbana: University of Illinois Press.

Dweck, C. S. (1975). The role of expectations and attributions in the alleviation of learned helplessness. *Journal of Personality and Social Psychology, 31,* 674–685.

Dweck, C. S., & Elliot, E. S. (1983). Achievement motivation. In E. M. Hetherington (Ed.), *Handbook of child psychology* (Vol. 4). New York: Wiley.

Dweck, C. S., & Reppucci, N. D. (1973). Learned helplessness and reinforcement responsibility in children. *Journal of Personality and Social Psychology, 25,* 109–116.

Egeland, J. A., Gerhard, D. S., Pauls, D. L., Sussex, J. N., Kidd, K. K., Allen, C. R., Hostetter, A. M., & Housman, D. E. (1987). Bipolar affective disorder linked to DNA markers on chromosome 11. *Nature, 325,* 783–787.

Ellis, A. (1962). *Reason and emotion in psychotherapy.* New York: Stuart.

Engel, G. L. (1968). A life setting conducive to illness: The giving -up–given-up complex. *Annals of Internal Medicine, 69,* 293–300.

Erdelyi, M. H. (1985). *Psychoanalysis: Freud's cognitive psychology.* New York: Freeman.

Eysenck, H. J. (1988). Personality and stress as causal factors in cancer and coronary heart disease. In M. P. Janisse (Ed.), *Individual differences, stress, and health psychology.* New York: Springer-Verlag.

Fincham, F. D., & Cain, K. M. (1986). Learned helplessness in humans: A developmental analysis. *Developmental Review, 6,* 301–333.

Fox, B. H. (1978). Premorbid psychological factors as related to cancer incidence. *Journal of Behavioral Medicine, 1,* 45–133.

Freud, S. (1893). Miss Lucy R. In *Collected works* (Vol. 1). London: Hogarth.

Friedman, H. S., & Booth-Kewley, S. (1987). The "disease-prone personality": A meta-analytic view of the concept. *American Psychologist, 42,* 539–555.

Friedman, M., & Rosenman, R. (1974). *Type A behavior and your heart.* New York: Knopf.

Friedman, M., Thoreson, C. E., Gill, J. J., Powell, L. H., Ulmer, D., Thompson, L., Price, V. A., Rabin, D. D., Breall, W. S., Dixon, T., Levy, R., & Bourg, E. (1984). Alteration of Type A behavior and reduction in cardiac recurrences in post myocardial infarction patients. *American Heart Journal, 108,* 237–248.

Friedmann, E., Katcher, A. H., Lynch, J. J., & Thomas, S. A. (1980). Animal companions and one-year survival of patients after discharge from a coronary care unit. *Public Health Reports, 95,* 307–312.

Fuller, R. C. (1989). *Alternative medicine and American religious life.* New York: Oxford University Press.

Gallagher, W. (1988, April). The DD's: Blues without end. *American Health,* pp. 80–88.

Gamzu, E. R. (1974). Learned laziness in pigeons. *The Worm Runner's Digest, 16,* 86–87.

Gardner, H. (1983). *Frames of mind: The theory of multiple intelligences.* New York: Basic Books.

Gardner, H. (1985). *The mind's new science: A history of the cognitive revolution.* New York: Basic Books.

Gavzer, B. (1988, September 18). Why do some people survive AIDS? *Parade Magazine,* pp. 4–7.

Gay, P. (1963). Introduction: The wit of Candide. In *Voltaire's Candide: A bilingual edition.* New York: St. Martin's Press.

Gibbs, N. (1989, July 31). Sick and tired. *Time,* pp. 48–53.

Gill, J. J., Price, V. A., Friedman, M., Thoreson, C. E., Powell, L. H., Ulmer, D.,

Brown, B., & Drews, F. R. (1985). Reduction in Type A behavior in healthy middle-aged American military officers. *American Heart Journal, 110,* 503–514.

Glass, D. C. (1977). *Behavior patterns, stress, and heart disease.* Hillsdale, NJ: Erlbaum.

Gochman, D. S. (1988). Assessing children's health concepts. In P. Karoly (Ed.), *Handbook of child health assessment: Biopsychosocial perspectives.* New York: Wiley.

Gordon, H. (1988). *Channeling into the New Age: The "teachings" of Shirley Mac-Laine and other such gurus.* Buffalo: Prometheus.

Gorman, J. (1989). Night of the living optimists. In *The man with no endorphins and other reflections on science.* New York: Penguin.

Gotlib, I. H., & Beatty, M. E. (1985). Negative responses to depression: The role of attributional style. *Cognitive Therapy and Research, 9,* 91–103.

Greenwald, A. G. (1975). Consequences of prejudice against the null hypothesis. *Psychological Bulletin, 82,* 1–20.

Hackett, T. P., & Cassem, N. H. (1974). Development of a quantitative rating scale to assess denial. *Journal of Psychosomatic Research, 18,* 93–100.

Hales, D., & Hales, R. E. (1987, November). Killing with kindness. *American Health,* pp. 61–65.

Heider, F. (1958). *The psychology of interpersonal relations.* New York: Wiley.

Hollon, S., & Beck, A. T. (1986). Research on cognitive therapies. In S. L. Garfield & A. E. Bergin (Eds.), *Handbook of psychotherapy and behavior change* (3rd ed.). New York: Wiley.

Holmes, T. H., & Rahe, R. H. (1967). The social readjustment rating scale. *Journal of Psychosomatic Research, 11,* 213–218.

House, J. S., Landis, K. R., & Umberson, D. (1988). Social relationships and health. *Science, 241,* 540–545.

House, J. S., Robbins, C., & Metzner, H. L. (1982). The association of social relationships and activities with mortality: Predictive evidence from the Tecumseh Community Health Study. *American Journal of Epidemiology, 116,* 123–140.

Ickes, W., & Layden, M. A. (1978). Attributional styles. In J. H. Harvey, W. Ickes, & R. F. Kidd (Eds.), *New directions in attribution research* (Vol. 2). Hillsdale, NJ: Erlbaum.

Jaret, P. (1986, June). Our immune system: The wars within. *National Geographic,* pp. 702–735.

Jaynes, G. D., & Williams, R. M. (Eds.) (1989). *A common destiny: Blacks and American society.* Washington, DC: National Academy Press.

Justice, B. (1988). *Who gets sick? How beliefs, moods, and thoughts affect your health.* Los Angeles: Tarcher.

Kalnins, I., & Love, R. (1982). Children's concepts of health and illness—and implications for health education: An overview. *Health Education Quarterly, 9,* 104–115.

Kamen, L. P., Seligman, M. E. P., Dwyer, J., & Rodin, J. (1987). Pessimism and cell-mediated immunity. Unpublished manuscript, University of Pennsylvania, described in M. E. P. Seligman, *Predicting depression, poor health, and presidential elections: A science and public policy seminar.* Washington, DC: Federation of Behavioral, Psychological, and Cognitive Sciences.

Kanner, A. D., Coyne, J. C., Schaefer, C., & Lazarus, R. S. (1981). Comparison of two modes of stress measurement: Daily hassles and uplifts versus major life events. *Journal of Behavioral Medicine, 4,* 1–39.

Kaplan, G. A., & Camacho, T. (1983). Perceived health and mortality: A nine-year follow-up of the human population laboratory cohort. *American Journal of Epidemiology, 11,* 292–304.

Karasek, R., & Theorell, T. (1990). *Healthy work: Stress, productivity, and the reconstruction of working life.* New York: Basic Books.

Kelley, H. H. (1973). The process of causal attribution. *American Psychologist, 28,* 107–128.

Kelly, G. A. (1955). *The psychology of personal constructs.* New York: Norton.

Kiecolt-Glaser, J. K., & Glaser, R. (1987). Psychosocial moderators of immune function. *Annals of Behavioral Medicine, 9,* 16–20.

King, N. J., Hamilton, D. I., & Murphy, G. C. (1983). The prevention of children's maladaptive fears. *Child and Family Behavior Therapy, 5,* 43–57.

Kobasa, S. C. (1979). Stressful life events, personality, and health: An inquiry into hardiness. *Journal of Personality and Social Psychology, 37,* 1–11.

Kobasa, S. C. (1982). Commitment and coping in stress resistance among lawyers. *Journal of Personality and Social Psychology, 42,* 707–717.

Kobasa, S. C., Maddi, S. R., & Courington, S. (1981). Personality and constitution as mediators in the stress-illness relationship. *Journal of Health and Social Behavior, 22,* 368–378.

Kobasa, S. C., Maddi, S. R., & Kahn, S. (1982). Hardiness and health: A prospective study. *Journal of Personality and Social Psychology, 42,* 168–177.

Krantz, D. S., Glass, D. C., & Snyder, M. L. (1974). Helplessness, stress level, and the coronary-prone behavior pattern. *Journal of Experimental Social Psychology, 10,* 284–300.

Kronfol, Z., & House, J. D. (1988). Immune function in mania. *Biological Psychiatry, 24,* 341–343.

Kushner, H. S. (1983). *When bad things happen to good people.* New York: Avon.

Lachman, M. E. (1988). *Personal control in later life: Implications for cognitive aging.* Invited address given at the Annual Meeting of the American Psychological Association, Atlanta.

Lachman, M. E. (1989). *When bad things happen to old people: Age differences in attributional style.* Unpublished manuscript, Brandeis University.

Langer, E. J. (1975). The illusion of control. *Journal of Personality and Social Psychology, 32,* 311–328.

Langer, E. J. (1978). Rethinking the role of thought in social interaction. In J. H. Harvey, W. Ickes, & R. F. Kidd (Eds.), *New directions in attribution research* (Vol. 2). Hillsdale, NJ: Erlbaum.

Langer, E. J. (1989). *Mindfulness.* Reading, MA: Addison-Wesley.

Lauzanne, S., & Wylie, I. A. R. (1931). American optimism: Pollyanna is dead. *Living Age, 340,* 605–606.

Lazarus, R. S. (1966). *Psychological stress and the coping process.* New York: McGraw-Hill.

Lazarus, R. S. (1979, June). Positive denial: The case of not facing reality. *Psychology Today,* pp. 44–60.

Lazarus, R. S. (1982). Thoughts on the relations between emotion and cognition. *American Psychologist, 37,* 1019–1024.

Lazarus, R. S. (1984). The costs and benefits of denial. In B. S. Dohrenwend & B. P. Dohrenwend (Eds.), *Stressful life events and their contexts.* New York: Prodist.

Lazarus, R. S., & Folkman, S. (1984). *Stress, appraisal, and coping.* New York: Springer.

Lefcourt, H. M. (1973). The functions of the illusions of control and freedom. *American Psychologist, 28,* 418–425.

Levine, G. F. (1977). "Learned helplessness" and the evening news. *Journal of Communication, 27,* 100–105.

Levy, S., Seligman, M. E. P., Morrow, L., Bagley, C., & Lippman, M. (1987). Survival hazards analysis in first recurrent breast cancer patients. Unpublished manuscript, University of Pittsburgh, described in M. E. P. Seligman, *Predicting depression, poor health, and presidential elections: A science and public policy seminar.* Washington, DC: Federation of Behavioral, Psychological, and ∖Cognitive Sciences.

Lin, E. H., & Peterson, C. (1989). [Explanatory style and coping with illness.] Unpublished data, University of Michigan.

Locke, E. A., Shaw, K. N., Saari, L. M., & Latham, G. (1981). Goal setting and task performance. *Psychological Bulletin, 90,* 125–152.

Locke, S., & Colligan, D. (1986). *The healer within: The new medicine of mind and body.* New York: New American Library.

Looney, D. S. (1987, July 6). The most happy fella. *Sports Illustrated,* pp. 28–29.

Maher, B. A., & Maher, W. B. (1979). Psychopathology. In E. Hearst (Ed.), *The first century of experimental psychology.* Hillsdale, NJ: Erlbaum.

Mahoney, M. J. (1974). *Cognition and behavior modification.* Cambridge, MA: Ballinger.

Maier, S. F. (1970). Failure to escape traumatic shock: Incompatible skeletal motor responses or learned helplessness? *Learning and Motivation, 1,* 157–170.

Maier, S. F., & Jackson, R. L. (1979). Learned helplessness: All of us were right (and wrong)—Inescapable shock has multiple effects. In G. H. Bower (Ed.), *The psychology of learning and motivation* (Vol. 13), New York: Academic Press.

Maier, S. F., Laudenslager, M., & Ryan, S. M. (1985). Stressor controllability, immune function, and endogenous opiates. In F. Bush & J. B. Overmier (Eds.), *Affect, conditioning, and cognition.* Hillsdale, NJ: Erlbaum.

Maier, S. F., & Seligman, M. E. P. (1976). Learned helplessness: Theory and evidence. *Journal of Experimental Psychology: General, 105,* 3–46.

Matthews, K. A. (1982). Psychological perspectives on the Type A behavior pattern. *Psychological Bulletin, 91,* 293–323.

McClelland, D. C. (1989). Motivational factors in health and disease. *American Psychologist, 44,* 675–683.

McCormick, R. A., & Taber, J. I. (1988). Attributional style in pathological gamblers in treatment. *Journal of Abnormal Psychology, 97,* 368–370.

McLeod, J. D. (1987). *Childhood parental loss and adult depression.* Unpublished doctoral dissertation, University of Michigan.

Meichenbaum, D. (1977). *Cognitive behavior-modification: An integrative approach.* New York: Plenum.

Melnechuk, T. (1985). Why has psychoneuroimmunology been controversial? *Advances, 2*(4), 22–38.

Meyer, D. (1980). *The positive thinkers.* New York: Pantheon Books.

Miller, W. R. (1983). Controlled drinking: A history and a critical review. *Journal of Studies on Alcohol, 44,* 68–83.

Mischel, W. (1979). On the interface of cognition and personality: Beyond the person-situation debate. *American Psychologist, 32,* 246–254.

Mischel, W., Ebbesen, E. B., & Zeiss, A. R. (1973). Selective attention to the self: Situational and dispositional determinants. *Journal of Personality and Social Psychology, 27,* 129–142.

Mossey, J. M., & Shapiro, E. (1982). Self-rated health: A predictor of mortality among the elderly. *American Journal of Public Health, 72,* 800–808.

Natapoff, J. N. (1982). A developmental analysis of children's ideas of health. *Health Education Quarterly, 9,* 130–141.

Nicholls, J. G. (1979). The development of perception of own attainment and causal attribution for success and failure in reading. *Journal of Educational Psychology, 71,* 192–197.

Nisbett, R. E., & Wilson, T. D. (1977). Telling more than we can know: Verbal reports on mental processes. *Psychological Review, 84,* 231–259.

Nolen-Hoeksema, S. (1986). *Developmental studies of explanatory style, and learned helplessness in children.* Unpublished doctoral dissertation, University of Pennsylvania.

Nolen-Hoeksema, S. (1987). Sex differences in unipolar depression: Theory and evidence. *Psychological Bulletin, 101,* 259–282.

Norem, J. K., & Cantor, N . (1986). Defensive pessimism: "Harnessing" anxiety as motivation. *Journal of Personality and Social Psychology, 51,* 1208–1217.

Oettingen, G., Seligman, M. E. P., & Morawska, E. (1988). *Pessimism across cultures.* Unpublished manuscript, University of Pennsylvania.

O'Leary, A. (1985). Self-efficacy and health. *Behaviour Research and Therapy, 23,* 437–451.

Ollendick, T. H. (1986). Child and adolescent behavior therapy. In S. L. Garfield & A. E. Bergin (Eds.), *Handbook of psychotherapy and behavior change* (3rd ed.). New York: Wiley.

Ornstein, R., & Sobel, D. (1984). *The healing brain.* New York: Simon & Schuster.

Ornstein, R., & Sobel, D. (1989). *Healthy pleasures.* Reading, MA: Addison-Wesley.

Overmier, J. B., & Seligman, M. E. P. (1967). Effects of inescapable shock upon subsequent escape and avoidance learning. *Journal of Comparative and Physiological Psychology, 63,* 23–33.

Park, J., & Sheff, V. (1989, August 28). Raiding *Cosby* for her stars, Debbie Allen turns *Pollyanna* into a black musical, *Polly! People Weekly,* pp. 102–104.

Parsons, J. E., & Ruble, D. N. (1977). The development of achievement-related expectancies. *Child Development, 48,* 1075–1079.

Pearlin, L. I. (1989). The sociological study of stress. *Journal of Health and Social Behavior, 30,* 241–256.

Peele, S. (1989). *The diseasing of America: Addiction treatment out of control.* Lexington, MA: Lexington Books.

Peirce, C. S. (1955). *The philosophical writings of Peirce* (J. Buchler, Ed.). New York: Dover.

Pelletier, K. R., & Herzing, D. L. (1988). Psychoneuroimmunology: Toward a mindbody model. *Advances, 5*(1), 27–56.

Pennebaker, J. W., Hughes, C. F., & O'Heeron, R. C. (1987). The psychophysiology of confession: Linking inhibitory and psychosomatic processes. *Journal of Personality and Social Psychology, 52*, 781–793.

Pennebaker, J. W., & O'Heeron, R. C. (1984). Confiding in others and illness rate among spouses of suicide and accidental-death victims. *Journal of Abnormal Psychology, 93*, 473–476.

Peterson, C. (1982). Learned helplessness and attributional interventions in depression. In C. Antaki & C. Brewin (Eds.), *Attributions and psychological change: A guide to the use of attribution theory in the clinic and classroom.* London: Academic Press.

Peterson, C. (1988a). *Explanatory style and academic performance.* Paper presented at the Annual Convention of the American Psychological Association, Atlanta, GA.

Peterson, C. (1988b). Explanatory style as a risk factor for illness. *Cognitive Therapy and Research, 12*, 119–132.

Peterson, C. (1991). The meaning and measurement of explanatory style. *Psychological Inquiry.*

Peterson, C., & Barrett, L. C. (1987). Explanatory style and academic performance among university freshmen. *Journal of Personality and Social Psychology, 53*, 603–607.

Peterson, C., & Bossio, L. M. (1989). Learned helplessness. In R. C. Curtis (Ed.), *Self-defeating behaviors.* New York: Plenum.

Peterson, C., Colvin, D., & Lin, E. H. (1989). *Explanatory style and helplessness.* Unpublished manuscript, University of Michigan.

Peterson, C., & Rosenwald, J. (1987). [Sigmund Freud's causal explanations.] Unpublished data, University of Michigan.

Peterson, C., Schulman, P., Castellon, C., & Seligman, M. E. P. (in press). The explanatory style scoring manual. In C. P. Smith (Ed.), *Handbook of thematic analysis.* New York: Cambridge University Press.

Peterson, C., & Seligman, M. E. P. (1984). Causal explanations as a risk factor for depression: Theory and evidence. *Psychological Review, 91*, 347–374.

Peterson, C., Seligman, M. E. P., & Vaillant, G. E. (1988). Pessimistic explanatory style is a risk factor for physical illness: A thirty-five year longitudinal study. *Journal of Personality and Social Psychology, 55*, 23–27.

Peterson, C., Semmel, A., von Baeyer, C., Abramson, L. Y., Metalsky, G. I., & Seligman, M. E. P. (1982). The Attributional Style Questionnaire. *Cognitive Therapy and Research, 6*, 287–299.

Peterson, C., & Stunkard, A. J. (1989). Personal control and health promotion. *Social Science and Medicine, 28*, 819–828.

Phillips, D. P., & Smith, D. G. (1990). Postponement of death until symbolically meaningful outcomes. *JAMA, 263*, 1947–1951.

Piaget, J. (1926). *The language and thought of the child.* New York: Harcourt, Brace.

Piaget, J. (1928). *Judgment and reasoning in the child*. New York: Harcourt, Brace.

Piaget, J. (1929). *The child's conception of the world*. New York: Harcourt, Brace.

Piaget, J. (1932). *Moral judgment of the child*. New York: Harcourt, Brace.

Piaget, J. (1950). *The psychology of intelligence*. New York: Harcourt, Brace.

Podmore, F. (1963). *From Mesmer to Christian Science: A short history of mental healing*. New Hyde Park, NY: University Books.

Porter, E. H. (1913/1938). *Pollyanna*. London: Harrap.

Portis, S. A. (1949). Idiopathic ulcerative colitis: Newer concepts concerning its cause and management. *JAMA, 139,* 208–214.

Prochaska, J. O., Velicer, W. F., DiClemente, C. C., & Fava, J. (1988). Measuring processes of change: Applications to the cessation of smoking. *Journal of Consulting and Clinical Psychology, 56,* 520–528.

Quine, W. V., & Ullian, J. S. (1978). *The web of belief* (2nd ed.). New York: Random House.

Rabkin, J. G., & Struening, E. L. (1976). Life events, stress, and illness. *Science, 194,* 1013–1020.

Radner, G. (1989, June). "I've fought so hard to live." *Redbook,* pp. 120–122, 160–164.

Ragland, D. R., & Brand, R. J. (1988a). Coronary heart disease mortality in the Western Collaborative Group Study: Follow-up experience of 22 years. *American Journal of Epidemiology, 127,* 462–475.

Ragland, D. R., & Brand, R. J. (1988b). Type A behavior and mortality from coronary heart disease. *The New England Journal of Medicine, 318,* 65–69.

Reifman, A., & Peterson, C. (1989). [Causal explanations by the Baltimore Orioles during the 1988 losing streak.] Unpublished data, University of Michigan.

Rokeach, M. (1971). Long-range experimental modification of values, attitudes, and behaviors. *American Psychologist, 26,* 453–459.

Rosen, G. M. (1987). Self-help treatment books and the commercialization of psychotherapy. *American Psychologist, 42,* 46–51.

Rosenhan, D. L., & Seligman, M. E. P. (1989). *Abnormal psychology* (2nd ed.). New York: Norton.

Rosenthal, R., & Rubin, D. B. (1982). A simple, general purpose display of magnitude of experimental effect. *Journal of Educational Psychology, 74,* 166–169.

Rothbaum, F., Weisz, J. R., & Snyder, S. S. (1982). Changing the world versus changing the self: A two-process model of perceived control. *Journal of Personality and Social Psychology, 42,* 5–37.

Ruble, D. N., Parsons, J. E., & Ross, J. (1976). Self-evaluative responses of children in an academic setting. *Child Development, 47,* 990–997.

Sagan, L. A. (1987). *The health of nations: True causes of sickness and well-being*. New York: Basic Books.

Scheier, M. F., & Carver, C. S. (1985). Optimism, coping, and health: Assessment and implications of generalized outcome expectancies. *Health Psychology, 4,* 219–247.

Scheier, M. F., & Carver, C. S. (1987). Dispositional optimism and physical well-being: The influence of generalized outcome expectancies on health. *Journal of Personality, 55,* 169–210.

Scheier, M. F., Matthews, K. A., Owens, J., Magovern, G. J., Lefebvre, R. C., Abbott, R. A., & Carver, C. S. (1989). Dispositional optimism and recovery from coronary artery bypass surgery: The beneficial effects on physical and psychological well-being. *Journal of Personality and Social Psychology, 57,* 1024–1040.

Schleifer, S. J., Keller, S. E., Siris, S. G., Davis, K. L., & Stein, M. (1985). Depression and immunity. *Archives of General Psychiatry, 42,* 129–133.

Sears, R. R., Maccoby, E. E., & Levin, H. (1957). *Patterns of child rearing.* Evanston, IL: Row, Peterson.

Seligman, M. E. P. (1973, January). Fall into helplessness. *Psychology Today,* pp. 43–48.

Seligman, M. E. P. (1974). Depression and learned helplessness. In R. J. Friedman & M. M. Katz (Eds.), *The psychology of depression: Contemporary theory and research.* Washington, DC: Winston.

Seligman, M. E. P. (1975). *Helplessness: On depression, development, and death.* San Francisco: Freeman.

Seligman, M. E. P. (1988). *Why is there so much depression today? The waxing of the individual and the waning of the commons.* Invited lecture at the Annual Convention of the American Psychological Association, Atlanta.

Seligman, M. E. P., & Maier, S. F. (1967). Failure to escape traumatic shock. *Journal of Experimental Psychology, 74,* 1–9.

Seligman, M. E. P., Maier, S. F., & Peterson, C. (in press). *Learned helplessness.* New York: Oxford.

Seligman, M. E. P., Nolen-Hoeksema, S., Thornton, N., & Thornton, K. M. (1989). *Athletic achievement and explanatory style.* Unpublished manuscript, University of Pennsylvania.

Seligman, M. E. P., Peterson, C., Kaslow, N. J., Tanenbaum, R. L., Alloy, L. B., & Abramson, L. Y. (1984). Attributional style and depressive symptoms among children. *Journal of Abnormal Psychology, 83,* 235–238.

Seligman, M. E. P., & Schulman, P. (1986). Explanatory style as a predictor of productivity and quitting among life insurance agents. *Journal of Personality and Social Psychology, 50,* 832–838.

Seligman, M. E. P., Castellon, C., Cacciola, J., Schulman, P., Luborsky, L., Ollove, M., & Downing, R. (1988). Explanatory style change during cognitive therapy for unipolar depression. *Journal of Abnormal Psychology, 97,* 13–18.

Selye, H. (1956). *The stress of life.* New York: McGraw Hill.

Shankland, R. (1947, July). She was glad, glad, glad! *Good Housekeeping,* pp. 41, 184–185.

Shilling, L. E. (1984). *Perspectives on counseling theories.* Englewood Cliffs, NJ: Prentice-Hall.

Siegel, B. S. (1986). *Love, medicine, and miracles.* New York: Harper & Row.

Siegel, B. S. (1989). *Peace, love, and healing.* New York: Harper & Row.

Simpson, W. F. (1989). Comparative longevity in a college cohort of Christian Scientists. *JAMA, 262,* 1657–1658.

Skinner, B. F. (1983). Intellectual self-management in old age. *American Psychologist, 38,* 239–244.

Smith, D., Peterson, C., & Pintrich, P. (1989). [Explanatory style and learning strategies.] Unpublished data, University of Michigan.

Smith, E. M., Morrill, A. C., Meyer, W. J., & Blalock, J. E. (1986). Corticotropin releasing factor induction of leukocyte-derived immunoreactive ACTH and endorphins. *Nature, 321,* 881–882.

Sontag, S. (1979). *Illness as metaphor.* New York: Vintage Books.

Sontag, S. (1988). *AIDS and its metaphors.* New York: Farrar, Straus, & Giroux.

Spiegel, D., Bloom, J. R., Kraemer, H. C., & Gottheil, E. (1989). Effect of psychosocial treatment on survival of patients with metastatic breast cancer. *Lancet, 109,* 888–891.

Sternberg, R. J. (1985). *Beyond IQ: A triarchic theory of human intelligence.* Cambridge: Cambridge University Press.

Stipek, D. J. (1981). Children's perceptions of their own and their classmates' ability. *Journal of Educational Psychology, 73,* 404–410.

Stroebe, M. S., & Stroebe, W. (1983). Who suffers more? Sex differences in health risks of the widowed. *Psychological Bulletin, 93,* 279–301.

Stroebe, W., & Stroebe, M. S. (1987). *Bereavement and health: The psychological and physical consequences of partner loss.* Cambridge: Cambridge University Press.

Suls, J., & Mullen, B. (1981). Life events, perceived control, and illness: The role of uncertainty. *Journal of Human Stress, 7,* 30–34.

Sweeney, P. D., Anderson, K., & Bailey, S. (1986). Attributional style in depression: A meta-analytic review. *Journal of Personality and Social Psychology, 50,* 974–991.

Taylor, R. B., Denham, J. R., & Ureda, J. W. (1982). *Health promotion: Principles and clinical applications.* Norwalk, CT: Appleton-Century-Crofts.

Taylor, S. E., & Brown, J. D. (1988). Illusion and well-being: A social psychological perspective on mental health. *Psychological Bulletin, 103,* 193–210.

The Sporting News (1989, June 19), p. 28.

Tillmann, W. A., & Hobbs, C. E. (1949). The accident-prone automobile driver: A study of the psychiatric and social background. *American Journal of Psychiatry, 106,* 321–331.

Tolle, S. W., Bascom, P. B., Hickam, D. H., & Beson, J. A. (1986). Communication between physicians and surviving spouses following patient deaths. *Journal of General Internal Medicine, 1,* 309–314.

Vaillant, G. E. (1977). *Adaptation to life.* Boston: Little, Brown.

Vaillant, G. E. (1983). *The natural history of alcoholism.* Cambridge, MA: Harvard University Press.

Vanden Belt, A. (1989). *Parental attributional style and its relationship to disabled and able-bodied children's classroom performance.* Unpublished honors thesis, University of Michigan.

van Doornen, L. J. P., & van Blokland, R. (1987). Serum-cholesterol: Sex specific psychological correlates during rest and stress. *Journal of Psychosomatic Research, 31,* 239–249.

Van Egeren, L. F. (1979). Social interactions, communication, and the coronary-prone behavior pattern: A psychophysiological study. *Psychosomatic Medicine, 41,* 2–18.

Verbrugge, L. M. (1989). Recent, present, and future health of American adults. In L. Breslow, J. E. Fielding, & L. B. Lave (Eds.), *Annual review of public health* (Vol. 10). Palo Alto, CA: Annual Review.

Watson, J. S. (1977). Depression and the perception of control in early childhood. In

J. G. Schulterbrandt & A. Raskin (Eds.), *Depression in childhood: Treatment and conceptual models.* New York: Raven.

Weidner, G., & Andrews, J. (1983). Attributions for undesirable life events, Type A behavior, and depression. *Psychological Reports, 53*, 167–170.

Weil, A. (1988). *Health and healing* (Rev. ed.). Boston: Houghton Mifflin.

Weinberger, M., Hiner, S. L., & Tierney, W. M. (1987). In support of hassles as a measure of stress in predicting health outcomes. *Journal of Behavioral Medicine, 10*, 19–31.

Weiner, B. (1986). *An attributional theory of motivation and emotion.* New York: Springer-Verlag.

Weiner, H. (1977). *Psychobiology and human disease.* New York: Elsevier.

Weisz, J. R. (1983). Can I control it? The pursuit of veridical answers across the life span. In P. B. Baltes & O. G. Brim (Eds.), *Life-span development and behavior* (Vol. 5). New York: Academic Press.

Weston, C. (1986, January). Are you a Pollyanna or a pessimist? *Seventeen,* p. 42.

Wilkinson, S. R. (1988). *The child's world of illness.* Cambridge: Cambridge University Press.

Williams, B. (1967). Rene Descartes. In P. Edwards (Ed.), *The encyclopedia of philosophy* (Vol. 2). New York: Macmillan.

Wong, P. T. P., & Weiner, B. (1981). When people ask "why" questions, and the heuristics of attribution search. *Journal of Personality and Social Psychology, 40*, 649–663.

Woodruff-Pak, D. (1988). *Psychology and aging.* Englewood Cliffs, NJ: Prentice-Hall.

Wortman, C. B. (1975). Some determinants of perceived control. *Journal of Personality and Social Psychology, 31*, 282–294.

Wortman, C. B., & Silver, R. C. (1989). The myths of coping with loss. *Journal of Consulting and Clinical Psychology, 57*, 349–357.

Yankelovich, D., & Gurin, J. (1989, March). The new American dream. *American Health,* pp. 63–67.

Yetman, N. R. (1970). *Voices from slavery.* New York: Holt, Rinehart, & Winston.

Zullow, H. M. (1988). [Personal communication.]

Zullow, H. M., Oettingen, G., Peterson, C., & Seligman, M. E. P. (1988). Pessimistic explanatory style in the historical record: CAVing LBJ, presidential candidates, and East versus West Berlin. *American Psychologist, 43*, 673–682.

Name Index

Subject Index